Praise for *Jesse*

"This book will break your heart. This book will make you angry. It will make you laugh and cry and cheer. But mostly, this book will lift you up."

—Ann Hood, author of
Comfort and *The Knitting Circle*

"This book made me laugh and cry and then laugh again until I was crying with laughter. Tough, tenacious, and fall-down funny: those words reflect the author's approach to life and the incredible talent of her magnificently smart and totally engaging son, Jesse. This kid's journey is one of a kind, and so is this book."

—Denis Leary, author of
Why We Suck and cocreator of *Rescue Me*

"*Jesse* is an incandescent memoir, glowing with a mother's love for her disabled son and fueled by her righteous anger. With fierce honesty and unexpected humor, Marianne Leone illuminates the challenges of Jesse's life, the courage with which he faced them, and the joy he brought those lucky enough to know him."

—Tom Perrotta, author of
The Abstinence Teacher and *Little Children*

"In prose so full of life and love and rage and grace it will fill the room where you read this book, Marianne Leone tells the story of her son, Jesse, a boy with cerebral palsy, a beautiful boy—brave, smart, funny, and determined to live his life as part of society, not segregated from it. Armed with a ferocious love, his parents set out to make sure Jesse has that chance. Here is a book in which sorrow and joy are found in the same breath, where ignorance is revealed to be indistinguishable from cruelty, but where grace abounds and justice finally triumphs. This is a love story, and a family story, and at its heart is the boy. Jesse died young, but he lives in these pages. I am grateful to have met him here."

—Abigail Thomas, author of
A Three Dog Life

"I was stunned. Stunned and moved to tears. This book is about unwavering courage, unbounded love, and perseverance in the face of adversity. It grabs you by the lapels and takes you on a wondrous, inspiring journey. I couldn't put it down and I now carry Jesse's journey in my heart."

—William H. Macy

"*Jesse* is an important book for any parent to read. No one should have to struggle the way the Coopers did for their beloved son. Their story forces us to imagine ourselves in their shoes, and to face the hard question of whose responsibility it is to speak for children who cannot speak for themselves."

—Richard Russo, author of
That Old Cape Magic

"Like a master tightrope walker, Marianne Leone avoids any fall here into understandable sentimentality or self-pity. Instead, she has stepped nakedly into the larger human truths of her own story and given us back a life-sustaining feast. *Jesse* goes beyond a living portrait of this remarkable boy and his family; it explores the unbreakable blood ties between parents and children, that chosen thread between husbands and wives, and that sometimes hazardous web of other people called bureaucracy. At the heart of all this is a Sufi aphorism that speaks agelessly to the true nature of loss itself, that it has an afterlife where spirit lies. With humor, guts, and grace, *Jesse* will carry you compellingly to yours!"

—Andre Dubus III, author of
House of Sand and Fog

"Heartbreaking, uplifting . . . but never, ever saccharine. . . . [A] fine and moving book."

—Steve Oney, *Los Angeles Times*

"*Jesse* is heartbreaking and honest. It's also funny, fierce and illuminating . . . You have to get this."

—Lauren Beckham Falcone, *The Boston Herald*

"Leone's character sketches are deft and humorous, and included throughout are selections of Jesse's poetry and photographs of the boy with family and friends, attesting to a life that, though short and often painful, was filled with accomplishment, love and joy."

—*Kirkus Reviews*

"Angry and loving, bitter and funny and, above all, honest, the emotion in this book is too alive to think of it as a memoir."

—John Sayles, writer/director of *Lone Star* and *Amigo*

"Actress, author, and 'running Madonna' Marianne Leone brings to the pages of *Jesse* what we strive for on the stage: truth, passion, humor, and soul that inhabits every moment."

—Wynn Handman, cofounder and artistic director of The American Place Theatre

"Jesse was an extraordinary individual who packed ten lifetimes into seventeen years. He had a great intellect and could envision life beyond the challenges of disability with poetry, dreams, and very real desires. But perhaps his greatest gift was in the way he taught so many in his community how to live with joy in the moment. Marianne puts the music from her son's heart into words. She brings us into her home, and won't let us go until we are inspired by the love her family shared."

—Ross Lilley, Executive Director, AccesSportAmerica

"With the gritty honesty of an outraged mother, *Jesse* tells of Marianne's family's pursuit of justice through hope, courage, and love."

—Rich Robison, Executive Director,
Federation for Children with Special Needs

"*Jesse* is wonderfully written, and is the legacy Jesse deserves. It is a gift to our community."

—Mindy L. Aisen, MD, Medical Director,
Cerebral Palsy International Research Foundation

"Marianne's beautiful prose mirrors the beauty of her unconditional love for Jesse. Jesse comes alive in the pages of the book in a way that reveals his grace and intelligence. I came to know and appreciate Jesse for the wonderful kid that he was. I also came to know Marianne and her husband, Chris, not only as advocates for Jesse and their family but as role models for what parents should do to protect and love their children."

—Michael Carroll,
founder of Romanian Children's Relief

Jesse

A Mother's Story

MARIANNE LEONE

SIMON & SCHUSTER PAPERBACKS
New York London Toronto Sydney

Simon & Schuster Paperbacks
A Division of Simon & Schuster, Inc.
1230 Avenue of the Americas
New York, NY 10020

First Simon & Schuster trade paperback edition April 2011

Previously published in hardcover as *Knowing Jesse*

SIMON & SCHUSTER PAPERBACKS and colophon are registered trademarks of Simon & Schuster, Inc.

For information about special discounts for bulk purchases, please contact Simon & Schuster Special Sales at 1-866-506-1949 or business@simonandschuster.com.

The Simon & Schuster Speakers Bureau can bring authors to your live event. For more information or to book an event, contact the Simon & Schuster Speakers Bureau at 1-866-248-3049 or visit our website at www.simonspeakers.com.

Designed by Nancy Singer

Manufactured in the United States of America

10 9 8 7 6 5 4 3 2 1

Library of Congress Cataloging-in-Publication Data

Leone, Marianne.
    Jesse : a mother's story / Marianne Leone.
        p. cm.
    1. Leone, Marianne.   2. Leone, Jesse, 1987–2005.   3. Mothers and sons—United States—Biography.   4. Cerebral palsied children—United States—Biography.   5. Cerebral palsied children—Family relationships.   6. Parental grief—United States.   I. Title.
CT275.L3676A3 2010
618.92'8360092—dc22   2010003446

ISBN 978-1-4391-8392-2
ISBN 978-1-4391-8432-5 (pbk)
ISBN 978-1-4391-8416-5 (ebook)

To Chris, my partner on the road
To Jesse, who is still lighting the way

Jesse

Prologue

All summer and fall I had been troubled by a dream I couldn't interpret. My mother, who had died that spring, appeared as a silent sentinel dressed in white, seated next to a café table covered by snowy linen on which one small candle burned. Like a sphinx, her face was inscrutable but not disapproving. She was eerily still and seemed drained of the passions that inflamed her in life—the hardwired resentments, the black humor that saw death lurking around every corner and met it with a sneer, a laugh, and a *vaffunculo.*

The candle tipped over and fell behind the table. I reached for it and the candle disappeared, falling through a hole in the floor that magically revealed the candle lighting millions of others. The light grew into a conflagration that did not harm but instead inspired awe in its magnitude, intensifying until the entire dream universe became a white-hot void.

The dream finally made sense on the morning of January 3, 2005, when I went in to wake up my son for school and found him dead in his bed. Everything in my universe was blotted out.

Journal, spring 1989: *"Someday I know I'll find him dead in his bed."*

How did I know this? I just knew. When I saw him lying there like a sleeping prince, his beautiful full lips tinged blue, I knew. I knew when I pulled up his eyelids and saw his huge brown eyes fixed and staring, I knew when I screamed for his father and watched him give CPR. And when he said, "Call nine-one-one," I knew. My son was wearing his T-shirt that read *"Anime fiammagente"*—souls aflame.

Jesse's small flame had joined the many.

The fates lobbed a medicine ball at my chest that January morning, and it's still lodged there, covering my heart in the spot where Jesse used to rest his head. It's hard and unyielding, too, the way his head would jackhammer against my chest during a seizure. Jesse had severe cerebral palsy and could not speak. He was also a straight-A student, a sophomore at his public high school who wrote poetry on his computer, aced every one of his Latin tests, and windsurfed in the summer.

That many people only saw Jesse's disabilities adds another dimension to grief, a surreal aspect to the isolation of my new altered state. Their perception is "It's for the best," or "He's free now, and so are you." But I would have gladly hefted Jesse's undersized frame for as long as my own body could tolerate the weight, and beyond, into my own infirm old age. My husband, Chris, and I used to joke that if we were to appear on an afternoon talk show, the legend at the bottom of the TV screen would read, "Tragic parents of severely handicapped child." But that's not how it was.

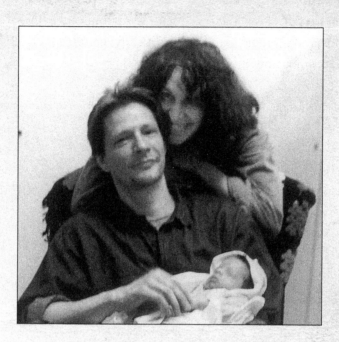

Jesse's first day home from the neonatal
intensive care unit, December 8, 1987

"My family is fancy ..."
—*Jesse Cooper*

CHAPTER ONE

"We Are Family"

Jesse, on the first anniversary of your death, you gave me a sign.

For Christmas and New Year's, your father and I had gone to southern Italy, where my memories of family were only ancestral and Chris's didn't exist at all. We stayed in a five-hundred-year-old palazzo in Naples, sleeping entombed in a high-ceilinged room with huge wooden shutters that covered the windows and blocked out noise from below. One tall window fronted the pedestrian street and the other opened onto a narrow Neapolitan alleyway.

I staggered out of bed, propelled by my body's memory of finding you last year, my mind not yet fully conscious. I opened the shutters, then a window. As I turned back to the room, I saw my laptop's dark screen come aglow all by itself. My screen saver is a picture of us laughing by the bay. You, in your little red jogging stroller, mouth wide open in a scream of delight. My mouth mirroring yours, your father's face suffused with joy. Goody, the little bichon frise, just happy to be included.

Before I could register that strangeness, the song "We Are Family" blared up from the street. I caught my breath; it was as loud as if the music was emanating from our walls. "Never Can Say Goodbye" followed, at the same volume. The wall of sound stopped at the end of the song. Then the everyday street sounds of Naples filtered up at a normal level, accordion music, shoppers' feet clacking over the cobblestones. Released from my enchantment, I looked over at Chris lying immobile on the bed. I didn't dare ask if he'd heard. But I knew he had.

You know why I knew it was you? It was the disco music in this ancient place that so perfectly expressed your sly humor, your mischief; the whiff of teenage irony in that choice of song. I can still see your Elvis lip curled, fighting a smile, as your crazy mother twirls you in your wheelchair to "I Will Survive."

We almost didn't have you at all. There we were, living out the New York starving-actor cliché, six flights up in the middle of Hell's Kitchen in a cacophony of neuron-grating sounds from the parking lot across the street and the fire station down the block. Air horn blasts from trucks routinely suspended conversation, and our answering machine informed callers that they had reached downtown Beirut.

Rushing to auditions early in the morning, I would see hookers already performing their craft in the alleyway next to the apartment building, and at night we watched adolescent boys selling themselves to businessmen on the corner. Homeless men camped on our doorstep in a nest of rags and news-papers. Even surrounded by sleaze, we were blissfully happy, with a gaggle of good friends struggling just like us amid the thrumming excitement of life in a world-class city. When the car alarms got too insistent we threw water balloons at them; we grew basil and mint on our fire escape and sojourned on the roof for brief vacations from the sensory overload of the street.

I pushed it. I waited until it was almost too late. I went to a psychic because I was afraid if I had a baby, the child and I would die.

But everything was fine. I kept a careful, almost obsessive record of everything I ate. I quit smoking. I never had a drink, even when we traveled to Italy, where wine is regarded as medicinal. I had amniocentesis because I was, in insulting medical terms, an "elderly primagravida." We saw you on the sonogram that day, your back turned to us as you lounged on your salty waterbed, your sex hidden. We knew you were a boy. You were Jesse La-nier, named after your great-grandfather. Before you were born, your name was Noonootz—your father is great at nicknames.

Jane Fonda and I and a herd of pregnant women did ex-ercises every day. I climbed flights and flights of stairs, walked with my arms crossed over you when I traversed the jangly streets of New York, and worked every day writing copy for MGM Home Video.

I was in my twenty-ninth week of a happily uneventful pregnancy and it was autumn in New York, that most sublime of seasons. We had just rented an apartment in Hoboken for November and had two months to get ready for your New Year's arrival.

Then, on Sixth Avenue, a man committed suicide by jumping out of a window at the Hotel Warwick. Walking to work, I arrived on the scene just in time to see the police drawing a blanket over his shattered head. A cop directed me to walk in the street. I looked down. The dead guy's brains were on my shoes. I started to hyperventilate. When I got to MGM I called Chris and asked him to come and get me.

I put the event out of my mind, or tried to, reassuring myself that I was strong, that pregnant women lived through wars and terrorism every day. That worked for about as long as it took to think it. The endless loop in my brain kept replaying that if I had walked a little faster to work that day, that hour, the man would've landed on you and me and not the sidewalk.

A week later, my immune system shut down and you were born. October 15, 1987, 2:52 p.m., ten weeks early, 3.7 pounds; you were born alive, born without drugs, born crying, breathing on your own, a tiny, perfect homunculus.

Your birth is as much a mystery to the medical establishment as your death. They suspected placenta abruptio, where the placenta suddenly tears away from the amniotic sac, but tests determined it wasn't that. Or maybe it was the high fever I had the night before. But there are no medical terms for "a guy jumps out of a window at the Hotel Warwick, almost lands on mother and child, mother has high fever a week later, and gives birth ten weeks early." Your death was determined to be "sudden unexplained death in epilepsy," a term so cruelly nonsensical it might as well have been "fickle finger of fate."

After your birth they took you away, and I didn't hold you

for almost two months. You belonged to the nurses, the neonatologist, the neurologist, the pediatrician. You lived with them in the neonatal intensive care unit, hooked up to tubes, your tiny body blurrily opaque through the plastic surrounding you. The tubes were connected to incomprehensible machines that were checked by sleep-deprived interns and residents who rarely deigned to acknowledge my presence. For seven weeks I watched your neighbor babies, undersized infants born on crack, shuddering in their isolettes. *Isolette:* the word makes me cringe, even now—the prettified, French-sounding "ette" at the end of a word describing a plastic cage that isolated you from me.

On the third day of your life, you had a massive cerebral hemorrhage, and they didn't expect you to last the week. We staggered like zombies back and forth from St. Vincent's Hospital in the Village to our walk-up in Hell's Kitchen. Chris and I sat glazed in front of episodes of *thirtysomething.* Onscreen, yuppies whined, "What if Janey isn't pretty?" as they peered into their baby's overdecorated crib. We threw things at the television and howled our despair, beyond tears.

Every day I scrubbed up and put on ceremonial cotton robes just to see you in your plastic coffin, like an enchanted prince. Every day I repeated the mantra "You're home, you're with us," crooning, cajoling, until you decided to stay, and you filled in like a developing photograph.

Deciding to stay was the first of your warrior choices. Those days, I walked around with a scream in my brain like a defective car alarm as I imagined the pain you must have been suffering. Daily spinal taps, tubes in every orifice, glaring lights, screeching beeps from all the sensors—I finally understood on a cellular level the impulse to offer up my own life to save someone else's. I wanted to take your pain. I wanted you to be free. I wanted to hold you, unfettered by plastic.

On December 8, 1987, you reached the magic six-pound bar and they let us take you home to Hoboken. Your diagnosis? Uncertain. Probably cerebral palsy. Maybe mental retardation. Maybe blind. Maybe deaf. Developmental delays. Seizure disorder, possibly. But you were home. Chris and I entered a state of euphoria that could not be dimmed by sleep deprivation, diaper changing, or any of the millions of parental tasks dealing with newborns. You were home. You were with us. I wore you in a sling all day and your pretty bassinet went unused at night. My mother, jealous by nature, carped, "You can't hold him all day long." Oh, yes. Yes, I could. Those months of heartbeat you missed out on would be supplied now. All day you were my kangaroo child. And at night, you lay on my chest sleeping. When you cried, Chris brought you to me and said, "He needs chest." But what he meant was that you needed to sync up your little iPod heart with mine.

But you still belonged to them, too. You belonged to the social worker at the Early Intervention Center who asked if I thought I was "overprotective"—one of the many occasions on which I suppressed hysterical, mad laughter as my reply. You belonged to the occupational therapist who fretted because Chris told her that we took you into our bed at night. This childless twentysomething informed us that such cuddling would "destroy our marriage." You belonged to the jocky, porcine orthopedist who wanted to cut your hamstrings to prevent your hip from someday dislocating. And you belonged to the neonatologist who wanted to have a shunt placed in your brain "for prophylactic reasons" and because your "clinical course might be better."

Those words snapped my leash. When I asked the neonatologist to tell me what she meant in plain English, she repeated that your "clinical course might be better," as if I hadn't heard her the first time. I knew that shunts were used to treat hydrocephalus, a swelling of the brain caused by a blockage of cerebrospinal fluid. But though your brain ventricles were enlarged, the fluid wasn't blocked. What help would the shunts be? I kept asking the doctor what she meant by "clinical course." Would you be unable to walk without this operation? Would you be mentally challenged? Would you die?

I asked her too many questions. Exasperated, she finally exclaimed, "Oh, Mrs. Cooper, it's only a piece of plumbing!" *Plumbing.* This was her casual, jokey description for an operation that would cut into your brain and insert a tube to drain into your stomach cavity. An operation that would require "revisions," euphemistic medspeak for many, many more operations as you grew. An operation that would leave you in danger of serious infections and more brain damage. And it was an operation you didn't need, we learned after getting a second opinion.

This was the first time I had to be physically restrained from attacking one of your "healers."

No wonder I had a recurring dream that you were frozen inside a block of ice. I would be wheeling you down an urban street in an expensive English pram that we couldn't afford in real life, and I would look down and you would be under a foot of clear, impenetrable ice. Your eyes were open. You were helpless. The dream would then morph into standard horror movie fare: screaming with no sound coming out, frantic digging at the ice, my limbs curiously moving in slo-mo, useless, ineffective. I would awake, chest heaving, and bolt from the bed to check on you. I would hover anxiously, not fully awake, over your sleeping body. In your sleep, you didn't look disabled. In your sleep, you belonged only to us.

▪

Later that day in Italy, one year after you died, we visited an echoey old church. We sat before a statue of the Madonna Addolorata, the Grieving Mother, in her august black robes, her polished wood face serene despite the seven swords piercing her heart. The swords represent her seven sorrows, which chronicle her Son's life and death, from Simeon's ominous prophecy at his birth to his untimely burial. I lit a candle for you and left your picture at her shrine. My face was serene, too, my swords invisible.

You were there. I heard you, disguised as an old Neapolitan praying out loud before a statue of San Francesco nearby. At the end of his prayer, the old man kissed his hand, gesturing to the saint, and making your sound for "yes."

"Yes. Yes. Yes. Yes."

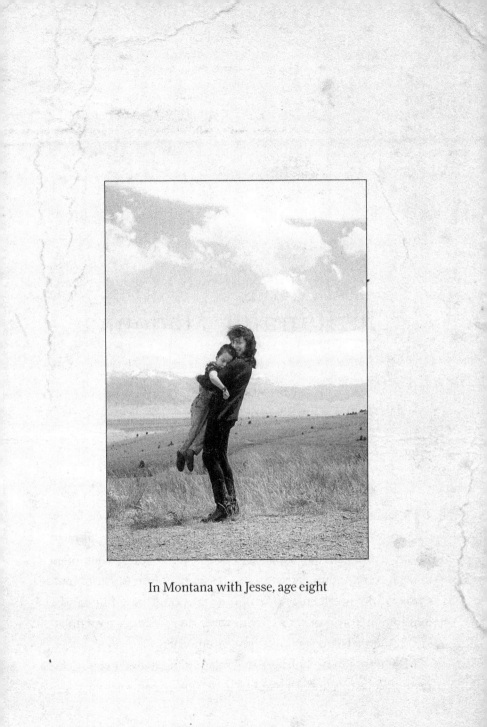

In Montana with Jesse, age eight

CHAPTER TWO

The Running Madonna

In the middle of the journey of our life
I found myself astray in a dark wood
Where the straight road had been lost sight of.
—*Dante*, Inferno

That first year after Jesse's death, all I want, all Chris wants, is to avoid the looming holidays at home, as if geographical distance and unfamiliar places will stopper years of memories and place us in an alternate, pre-Jesse, pain-free environment. Chris works fourteen-, fifteen-hour days on a new film, and I join him in Toronto, where I can work on revising a screenplay and pretend Thanksgiving is just another day.

But then I'm up before dawn, pacing the gilded cage of the posh hotel suite, and it's magical in an out-of-control Sorcerer's-

Apprentice kind of way. There are walls of glass, a dusting of snow on the streets below; a billboard that's eye level with me is lit up, its festive message—"Sick Kids and You"—glowing against the dim Toronto sky. The punch line underneath reads, "Equals Health," but I can't see that from here.

I sit for hours. I'm on the run, but only in my mind. I zig-zag across the memory minefields, losing ground every minute, every hour, every day.

The night before Jesse's memorial service I wrote an address that our friend Ross delivered the next day; we were incapable of moving our lips, standing up, addressing a crowd. The speech was high-flown, flowery, fervent. I wrote that parents of severely disabled children were "touched by the Divine." I said we had been transformed, offered a glimpse of the true secret of the universe, unconditional love. I quoted the Sufi poet Rumi: "This is love: to fly toward a secret sky, to cause a hundred veils to fall each moment. First, to let go of life. Finally, to take a step without feet." I said that Jesse had lifted us and made us fly, had caused the veils of prejudice to fall with just a smile, had taught us to let go of everything that distracts us from living life to the fullest, and finally that Jesse, who had never taken a step in his too short life, had led us to take many steps toward further understanding the love he brought to us.

Eleven months after his death, these words seem impossibly high-flown, composed, hopeful. Now I don't believe. I am not transformed. I can't love just anyone unconditionally. I can't transfer that light to someone by seeing Jesse in him or her. My compass no longer points to true north.

Everything I buy in Toronto tears—a pair of long black

stockings rip the first time I try them on, and a fleece glove splits along the seam of my middle finger, a symbolic gesture to this frozen tundra of a town where it's gray every single day. Everything is ripped apart in this purgatory of a place.

▣

That first year, I stumbled through the labyrinth that had grown up over the clear-cut path that had once been my life. Nothing was familiar. I tried to order my new world, to create a primer for the first year of grief in six not-so-easy lessons:

1. Avoid the local supermarket. Don't go to the mall. Do only essential errands and then only at odd hours. If you meet someone you know, run away before they say something that will irrationally enrage you.
2. To reenter the feeling world, start with symbols and archetypes. The cool painted face of the Virgin immobilized with pain, dressed like a great black-clad Barbie doll with seven swords in her heart. Let her be you for a while. Rest. Step back. Breathe in and out. Try to anchor your soul to your body before it blows away like fog on a marsh.
3. Decide you will swim in the bay, because it once gave you pleasure. Slide out of bed for the first time in days and combat-crawl until your body is upright. Stand before the bay and note with rising pleasure—joy!—the way the ocean's tang filters through nose, throat, lungs; the primal weightlessness of floating; the sun smoothing your up-turned face. But be aware: this release lasts only as long as

your body is buoyed by something else. Back on dry land, the gravity of loss brings the body back to its knees, bereft.
4. Realize that you don't want to reenter the feeling world: it hurts too much. You have no textbook for how to grieve.
5. Go back to step one. Start all over again. Look for signs. Look for signs everywhere. Create a whole new world.
6. Put the primer away. It doesn't teach you anything. You live in the labyrinth. It's your new home.

◼

I have to be careful when I talk about signs. Some people more pragmatic than I are tsk-tsking over the fact that I'm not on antidepressants. It's antisocial, even un-American, not to bury my grief. When your emotions are flatlined, at least you don't talk about signs. It's embarrassing to be a Pietà. People edge away from you in supermarkets, afraid your grief will taint them. You might cry. You might be "inappropriate." You might remind them that what is precious to them could be snatched away in a heartbeat.

In America, take the Xanax. It's the safest way.

When my father died, my un-American mother fainted, screamed, tried to pull him out of the casket, spat "Fuck God" at the nuns when they tried their platitudes on her. *Really embarrassing,* I thought then, squirming in my fifteen-year-old skin. Six months later, I had asthma and she didn't. I couldn't breathe at night. I lay sleepless in bed, my father's death and my own mortality on my chest like a rock. My mother, all in black, could breathe.

Of course, my mother's culture had icons, songs of lamentation, and dress codes for grief. She could turn to the Madonna Addolorata for consolation. She could put on black garb and sing *"Scura mae,"* a lament that means "You have left me dark." But, aside from the all-black wardrobe, which I already possess, I am too American for these rituals. I don't live in a culture that would recognize them anyway. My culture is miles away from grief, or aging, or even acknowledging the existence of death.

I invoke Jesse like an amulet, like a scapular, like a precious stone against the world and all its woes. I keep going back to Italy because that is where I found him.

◼

My sister and I stand among packed crowds in the Piazza Garibaldi in my mother's hometown of Sulmona on Easter morning, 2006. It is fifteen months since Jesse died. We are here to witness a transformation, to take part in an ancient ritual of rebirth we had heard about from our mother since childhood.

The Running Madonna—*La Madonna che scappa*—is a centuries-old Easter procession in Sulmona, a mountain town in southern Italy that is also famous for the production of *confetti*, the sugared almonds with which newlyweds are pelted as they leave the church.

Today, a statue of the Virgin Mary represents the Madonna Addolorata, the archetype of the grieving mother, a memento mori for all to see. She is dressed in black robes and held aloft by six strong men as she searches for her son.

I, too, am dressed in black. I have been the Madonna for a year and a half now, looking for my son in the places we visited during the happiest year of our lives, but I'm also looking for my mother in the place she grew up. I found her half sister, her *sorellastra*—a word the Italians told me not to use; it's cold, a denial of common blood. She lived in a lonely house at the foot of the fierce Apennines. A strange look-alike version of my mother, expunged of all resentment and anger, yet she embodied my mother's love with enveloping warmth, open arms, tears of joy and sadness. She held me and cried for Jesse, whom she had never met, and for me and for my loss. *La vita e bella e dura*—life is beautiful and hard.

But the crowd today, full of children and teenagers and young parents, is not solemn. They are giddy and the children clutch balloons. The crowd reminds me of revelers at Fenway Park; the statue of the Madonna at the other end of the piazza seems only incidental, like a body overlooked at a boisterous wake.

Statues of St. Peter and St. John knock on the door of the church three times. In the distance, the Madonna waits hesitantly, unbelieving. The door opens to reveal her Son standing there, risen from the dead, glorified. When the mother sees the son she thought she'd lost forever, she breaks into a frenzied run. Her black robes fly off. There is a collective gasp in the piazza. Underneath the black robes, the Madonna wears green, for *speranza,* hope.

With typical Italian overkill, the Hallelujah chorus blares over loudspeakers and twelve white doves fly out from under the Madonna's pedestal, underscored by firecrackers. I smile as tears spring to my eyes, and I think of my own mother, who described this spectacle to me with girlish awe, a memory of her own presence in this square so many years before.

■

I didn't find Jesse in the piazza that day. He might have been there for a brief moment, when a SpongeBob SquarePants balloon hovered blasphemously close to the Running Madonna. I thought of Jesse's teenage smirk, his love of teasing. But I didn't find him.

I'm running, running, trying to get these robes to fly off. I'm looking for my son.

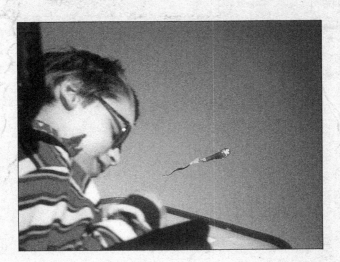

Jesse, age ten, on Plymouth Beach

My best dream is to fly
Soaring through the air
—*from Jesse's last poem, "I Am," 2004*

CHAPTER THREE

The Not-Jesse

My favorite aunt, Ellie, died four months after Jesse. She was the fun one, the one that I spent summers with as a kid, the one who let me stay up late and watch movies and eat onion rings, the one I called every day, the one I quoted to my friends because she was such a character. One of her lines even made it into my friend Nancy's movie *True Love*: "Uncle Benny and I saw that *Last Tangle in Paris*. Filthy! They showed the *bush*!"

Ellie and Benny were married for fifty-six years. The brutal week Ellie died, Uncle Benny never let go of her hand. Even after she left her ravaged body, he held her hand, muttering to her about trips not taken to Vegas and Aruba, deranged with love and loss. He died within the year. A young driver had overturned Benny's company truck and died instantly. When my uncle visited the scene, his heart, always too big for his stocky little frame, burst.

I stood over his body in the emergency room cubicle, the same room where Jesse had lain. I put my hand on the smooth top of his head. He was still warm and I heard him laughing. I saw him swimming up toward Ellie, legs pedaling in space, *Glad to be outta here*, as he would say.

So, in 2007, two years later, I feel like a female Job when I recount my recent history to strangers: my mother, Jesse, Ellie, Benny, all gone. They say, "Wow. I can't imagine it." Well, I couldn't, either. But what my brain couldn't comprehend, my body did: the visceral sadness was turning into something that I couldn't yet feel.

What I couldn't imagine was becoming not only imaginable but palpable, a thing with weight and mass and millions of blood vessels draining my strength, my energy, and my—by now—fading will to live. All year I had the strange sensation of being barely tethered to my body. It was as if I couldn't hear my actual body pain; it was being drowned out by the drumming soul pain of loss. A wise-ass genie appeared and granted my heart's desire: all those wishes that I could just disappear as they had started to come true. I got thinner and paler. I became a phantom, a shade.

Chris was away most of that year. He took three jobs in a row, wrapping the work around him like a magic cloak, submerging himself into three different characters. I envied him until I got a call from my on-again, off-again job with *The Sopranos*. For three seasons I played Joanne Moltisanti, the bitter, alcoholic mother of Christopher (played by Michael Imperioli) on the hit show about a Mafia boss and both of his extended families, the criminal one and the far more dangerous one related by blood.

After Jesse died, I had wondered whether someday I would reenact on national television the loss of a son. This wasn't idle speculation: on a mob show, people are always getting whacked. And this was the final season, where the body count could be in double digits by the third episode.

In November, I got the script. My television son was dead. The wake would take place on a set that re-created a typical Italian-American funeral home. I had no lines. The script called for me to walk toward the casket with my son in it, fall to my knees, and let out a wrenching primal scream.

A wrenching primal scream? Piece of cake for a female Job, right? Believe me, I had plenty of primal screams under my belt. But they were all expelled in the privacy of my home or in the thickly wooded conservation land where I walked Jesse's dog, Goody. In that lonely chapel of pine, my sobs and high-pitched screams were echoed only by a murder of crows. This reenactment would be on a brightly lit set with bored camera people standing around. Pieces of tape placed discreetly on the floor would tell me where I was to fall to my knees, overcome with grief. And there would be about three chances to get it right, or be frozen for posterity on film looking like I belonged in a Grade Z horror flick.

On the day of the shoot I was picked up at my hotel in midtown Manhattan and driven to Silvercup Studios in Queens, where the show was filmed. It was 5:30 a.m., and a queasy gray light was beginning to uncover the industrial landscape of Long

Island City. I headed for my dressing room, a tiny cubbyhole near the set with bare walls, a low sofa, and harsh lighting. I reported to the hair and makeup trailer, clutching my coffee, only to find that my naturally ravaged look was just perfect and I would need no makeup that day. Some of my friends on set knew about Jesse, but most of the actors and tech people did not.

I returned to my dressing room and started to prepare. I looked at pictures of Jesse, and began to let myself feel the loss, the emotion I daily held at bay like a dangerous clawed animal that appears out of nowhere in your dreams, intent on ripping your heart out of your chest. Now I called the beast, embraced it, let it consume me.

The first scene was simple. I was to be standing with my back to the camera, in front of the casket, leaning for support on an actor playing my boyfriend. The art department had the funeral home exactly right, down to the gaudy over-the-top floral arrangements. I walked onto the set and turned around and walked out, my knees suddenly weak. My mother, Ellie, and Benny had all been waked in a funeral home exactly like this one. The air was stifling, cloying with the scent of flowers; the set bustling with grips and electrics going about their business, arranging furniture, adjusting lights, marking actors' places on the floor. Wearing a long black dress and looking pale as the undead, I took my position for the first take. It was an establishing shot with no dialogue. After a short break we went into the second take, same shot. The lights seemed brighter, hotter.

Just before the third take I looked around the set, and my eyes settled on an arrangement that had a banner with gilt lettering: "Beloved Son." I woke up on the floor. A grizzled angel named Arthur had his fingers pressed into the pulse at my throat and was shouting, "You on meds?" an inch from my face. He was an ex–New York City cop now playing one of Tony Soprano's mob guys; years of conditioning had propelled him to action in an emergency situation. Now his handsome face loomed over me like an eclipsed moon, a baby Fresnel light behind him haloing his visage. I blinked at him, dazed. It had been a total blackout: no visions, no tunnel of light, no otherworldly chimes. Just merciful blackness. A hushed crowd stood around me, staring. Things got even more surreal when a tiny Asian woman, a helpful extra, told me that she was a dentist. But I didn't need a root canal. I needed to get through the next hours without fainting again.

When they finally got to my scene, at around ten o'clock that evening, we were at that stage in a long shoot when the crew is exhausted and cranky, and the extras and actors are joking around, bored out of their minds. I took my seat in front of the casket and desperately tried to shut out my surroundings, plugged into the iPod hidden away in my prop purse. I saw my friend Sharon Angela encouraging me from the sidelines, the lush features on her expressive face now taut with concern. She mouthed silently, *You're there. Just relax.* Michael Imperioli entered and climbed into the coffin, provoking more giggles among the actors. The director signaled me. I turned off the opening bars of "Calling All Angels," staggered to my feet, fell to my knees, and did the primal scream.

The actors applauded, and some had tears in their eyes. It felt shamanic, like I was channeling someone else, everyone else, all those mothers who had lost their children. It was a gift, a release. That night, in a dream that was not a dream, Jesse whispered in my ear, "I'm always with you."

What's hilarious in a get-over-yourself way is that the whole televised scene lasted eight seconds, if that. And I really didn't care. No, that's not true. I did care. The actor and writer parts of me had always coexisted with the mother of Jesse. The actor wanted to do justice to the scene. But the mother of Jesse just wanted to scream.

By December, I was weak, tired all the time, unable to eat, and had lost more than twenty-five pounds from my already slight frame. Chris was scared and urged me to see a doctor. I don't even have a primary physician, just an OB-GYN. Jesse's history of consistent, painful, even life-threatening mistakes in the world of mainstream medicine made me reluctant to have anything to do with those practitioners. I was getting through menopause with a witch's brew of herbs and acupuncture but now, obviously, nothing in the alternative medicine world was working.

I kept getting weaker and sicker. There was a dull pain in my stomach that worsened when I ate anything. I couldn't enjoy my morning coffee, or even my special vice, dark chocolate. I craved meat, but couldn't eat it. Nothing tasted right. Two years before I had lifted my eighty-five-pound son in and out of his wheelchair five times a day. Now I could barely lift his dog, who weighed ten pounds. I dreamed I was hurtling down a rickety staircase toward dark, churning water.

I made a call and, holding my nose, jumped into the doctor pool at Mass General.

It was cancer. A tumor that weighed what Jesse weighed at

birth. A three-and-a-half-pound Rorschach blot from the planet Rage 'n' Grief that clung to my upper intestines. My life was really in the balance. I wasn't afraid. I wanted to die, to see my son again. The pain would be gone forever, and the not-Jesse would be the entrance fee to seeing the real Jesse. And if I didn't see him, if it was really just lights out, blackness forever—well—I welcomed that, too. I never voiced any of these feelings, not to Chris, not to my family, not to friends. I hugged my secret wish for oblivion to myself as closely as I used to hold Jesse. I was weak, I was sick, and the world was receding. Good. There was nothing left in this world I wanted.

I met with the surgeon, the anesthesiologist; I took the pre-op stress test, I gave up vials of blood, but it was all happening to someone else, someone pretending to fight for her life.

My friend Maggie sat on the sofa in my hospital room on the twenty-second floor cutting out elements for her handcrafted valentines. She looked like the subject of an old-fashioned valentine herself, with her heart-shaped face, rosebud lips, and nimbus of curly black hair streaked with gray. Finished creations framed the large glass window overlooking Storrow Drive. For extra protection, she had festooned the entire room with Mexican banners depicting the Virgin of Guadalupe.

One of my oldest, dearest friends, Maggie was a film producer by trade and my personal savior over these past years of living dazedly. Not only had she and my friend Nancy "produced" Jesse's memorial service at a time when Chris and I were both mentally missing in action, she had spent the time since then reminding me that I was still alive and teaching me how to reactivate my senses. She took me white-water rafting, made me buy a bright orange dress, tempted me with succulent food, triggered uncontrollable laughter and tears, rubbed life in my face like a benevolent schoolyard bully. She was my protector before, during, and after the surgery that would remove the cancerous tumor shrouding my intestines.

The doctors weren't sure what they would find when they cut into me, if the cancer had spread, if the tumor was so entangled they would have to remove my intestines. I was too tired to care at this point. This vampire growth was taking my life, growing stronger as I weakened. The nurses kept pumping blood into me, hourly, until I received four pints, enough to sustain me through what could be a long surgery. Chris hovered nearby, his worry roiling him inward until he lost most of his ability to speak. Now he reeled like a punch-drunk fighter, his blue-gray eyes beseeching me to turn around and come back from my entranced shamble away from him.

I always see my son as a bird, a strong bird. A hawk. I saw Jesse circling overhead when a tree was dedicated to him outside the entrance to his high school. He swooped down over our deck when Chris and I were on the phone, working on the details of a donation to help spring forty disabled Romanian kids from an orphanage and into foster homes. He flew down low right before we left for Naples that first year, fleeing Christmas and its holly jolly mockery.

The hawk sightings had become my new religion. I was a solitary practitioner and didn't proselytize. Some had joined this new faith, but they were as crazy as I was.

So when I was on the twenty-second floor of Mass General in Boston waiting for them to take me downstairs to remove the Not-Jesse, I wasn't surprised when the hawk nearly slammed into the huge glass window of my hospital room, then stayed there flapping its wings to make sure I got Jesse's message: *I'm always with you.*

Then I was in a shadowy crypt with bodies on either side of me. A wounded beast was lowing, howling its death knell, and the sound permeated everything until I became the sound. I was the beast. Blackness swallowed me up again.

This was the recovery room, I would later realize.

When my eyes opened and I emerged from the haze, I saw Chris looming over me, beaming. He looked like a teen heartthrob, and Maggie popped in and out of the frame behind him like a giggling jack-in-the-box, repeating over and over, "It's good news! It's all good!" I mumbled to Chris, "You look twenty years younger."

It was good news—miraculous news, the surgeon told me. They had removed the Not-Jesse and there was no cancer anywhere else, not in any of my lymph nodes. They had reattached my intestines and, after recovery, I would be able to eat again, anything I wanted, even dark chocolate. They would follow my progress with blood tests and CT scans for the next few years, but I had been given a pass. I was going to live.

I think of the line from a Keats poem, "I have been half in love with easeful Death," and I realize now that loving Jesse and loving death are not the same thing. This love of easeful death is one more thing I have to give up. I am healthy. I am well, and the only reminder of this dance toward oblivion is a wavy twelve-inch scar in the middle of my stomach, which I love because it's a battle scar, and life won.

At least, if I can't touch you, Jesse, if I can no longer smooth back your cowlicky fine hair or unfurl your beautifully shaped fingers, or revel in your earthly beauty, I can still hear you and see you when you come to me.

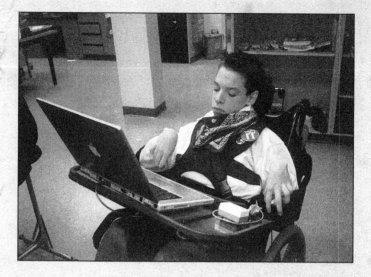

Jesse, age twelve, using his computer in middle school

Inside/Outside

On the inside, I walk

On the outside, I give

On the outside, I am mute

On the outside, I give

On the inside, I speak

On the inside, I walk

—*Jesse's first poem, age ten*

CHAPTER FOUR

"On the Outside,
I Am Mute"

The world is my book
I hear all its voices
—From Jesse's last poem, "I am"

Goody's huge black eyes trip my guilt sensors from a distance of twenty feet. His head swivels, assessing my every move like some coolly mad Dr. Frankenstein checking out his creation. He beams thoughts into my brain that become so insistent I am relieved that he has not yet willed me to shoot couples in cars. Ever since Goody, our twelve-year-old bichon frise, was diagnosed with congestive heart failure, I have been compelled by pity and fear to do his bidding. His paw imperiously strikes the snack drawer and I hover while he decides which snack stick he would like me to hold for him as he nibbles it delicately. Every morning he has me drive him to the parking lot of the local conservation area, where I stand and await his pleasure. Hang around and sniff car tires? Ramble among the weeds? Attempt a short walk? Whatever his choice, it's my duty to stand and walk a few paces behind. If I don't, he whips his head around, beaming those black eyes at me. It's all up to him, my ten-pound master. It's up to me to figure out what he's trying to tell me.

I fixate on Goody now the way I concentrated on Jesse then, my senses alert and tingling, trying to understand. But Goody's needs are a dog's needs, and his intellect is limited. Having a nonverbal child means learning to really look and listen. The rewards of nonverbal communication are as deep and subtle as the song of a whale, as complex and yearning as the trumpet of Miles Davis.

Goody is really Jesse's dog. He wanted a dog for so long, and when six-year-old Jesse sat on Santa's lap, all the neurons fired in his brain correctly, his synapses lighting up with sheer little-boy longing. Galvanized by the star power of Santa, Jesse was able to blurt out "Dog." Chris and I exchanged looks. It was three days before Christmas. "He's getting a dog," I said.

On Christmas morning, Goody appeared on Jesse's bed, a little white fluffball who looked more like a baby harp seal than a dog. Goody was, forever after, Jesse's canine sibling, obsessively licking his spastic closed fists, lying in the crook of his arm during therapy, sleeping with him, humping his leg in a brotherly bid for dominance, sprawled across his lap in the wheelchair while Jesse worked on his computer.

In my cruel and complacent youth, I made fun of people who talked funny, like my mother, or Joe "Me-do," the brain-damaged guy who was the church janitor and could only say "me-do" about his chores. In college, my friends and I all had roles in our pompous drama professor's vanity production, *Divinas Palabras* by Ramón del Valle-Inclán. One of the main characters is a "hydrocephalic idiot," who could only say "Guay, guay. Huagh." He was played by my friend Steve, in a giant plastic head that was replaced in the second act by a bloody dented head when I, in the role of his aunt, discovered him "Eaten! Eaten by pigs!" There's a picture of us backstage—Steve with his giant plastic head, me in my black garb and face paint—the two of us waving cigarettes with Noël Coward–like nonchalance to make the picture more absurd. Absurd, of course, because the world of "hydrocephalic idiots" who could only say "guay, guay" was as unreal to a bunch of nineteen-year-old college students as the grotesque characters in the play were.

Then Jesse came into my life, and I learned about how motor damage to the brain can interfere with the many muscles needed to speak. I learned to interpret Jesse's sounds, which were not "guay" or "huagh" but high-pitched screams of delight when he was a baby, and low, infectious chuckles when he got older, chuckles that escalated into belly laughs and deepened his child voice into a future man's voice I hear only in my dreams. I learned that even though the light of intelligence burned through Jesse's entire being, a nonverbal child has to prove that he's not an "idiot" to the world again and again and again.

Speaking in words isn't always communication, of course. There can be a definite disconnect from mouth to brain even in people without Jesse's brain injury. If you don't believe me, turn on the television and listen to the political pundits and talk show hosts, bloviators with perfectly functional mouth-to-brain muscles who roar and snarl like beasts, saying nothing at all.

Words were meaningless when I took basic acting classes in New York. I was taught to ignore the words and to answer only what I heard *under* the words. My class did hours of repetition exercises, facing each other, repeating senseless phrases: "You have blue eyes." "I have blue eyes." "You have blue eyes." "I have blue eyes." We did this until we could hear what was under the words and answer truthfully to the tone, the real emotion behind the meaningless words. Our teacher slouched in a folding chair and chewed on a coffee stirrer. If we hesitated to respond during the exercise he would bark out, "Answer that." Sometimes the exercise would end in both parties collapsing in helpless laughter; more often, anger would creep in and escalate to shouting, as if rage were the essential core of communication. Chris studied the same method with a different teacher. What Chris and I didn't know then was that we were in basic training for Jesse, and that the core of our communication with Jesse was powered by something else, driven by a hunger to know him, like the hunger that drives mystics to know God.

I knew Jesse was intelligent. I didn't need words to know that. I knew it when he was eight months old, when he burst out laughing the first time he heard the squeaky voices of the Chipmunks singing a Christmas song. He laughed at other silly jokes, too, things that make any baby hysterical, fishy faces and fart sounds. He became entranced with his own voice and we would laugh with delight to hear him respond to a question with a full-force yell, like a baby marine. He wore a smirk the whole time our yelling game went on, letting us know he was in on the prank. He understood us, even when he couldn't form the words to reply.

We had even heard him attempt "I love you" and other words. I told this to his pediatric neurologist when Jesse was around four, after he gave Jess an exam on our first (and last) visit to him. The neurologist looked at me with distaste. I was being deliberately obtuse, wasting his time with wishful thinking. I was obviously "in denial." From his Olympian neurological heights, the doctor pronounced his solemn verdict: Jesse would never be "intellectually normal." He said this to Chris and me, in front of Jesse. Then he asked, with what his lizard brain no doubt thought was kindness, if we planned to have more children. Chris wept on the way home as Jesse slept in my arms, and asked me what the neurologist meant by that, about having more children. "Get a good one," I said. "A different one." I looked down at Jesse's tufted teddy-bear hair. I wanted this one.

The very next week, Jesse worked with his occupational therapist on his shapes puzzle. Chris had glued wooden knobs to the shapes so Jess could grasp them easily. The therapist asked for the rectangle, then the square. It took Jess a full minute to tame his wavering arm to grasp each piece, but he delivered each shape correctly. Then she asked for the octagon. Instead of reaching for the shape, Jesse said, with great intensity: "Oct . . . eight." I heard him say it, and thanked all the fates that the therapist heard it, too, so I wouldn't get any more "in denial" looks when I reported this feat to other medical doubting Thomases. I told Chris that I knew teenagers who didn't know an octagon had eight sides. As far as I was concerned, our son was brilliant and we would raise him that way.

"Screw the itsy bitsy spider," I said. "Let's give him Yeats."

Years later, when his intelligence was finally tested correctly, using an adapted computer, Jesse scored in the ninety-ninth percentile. I wrote to the neurologist, that ice-cold genius who didn't know the basics of human compassion. I told him that I knew how hard it must be for him not to confuse himself with God, since he had acolyte interns hanging on his every word and parents praying to him for answers, but that he was most definitely not God. In fact, he was a murderer. He murdered the futures of brain-damaged children every day by making absurd hubristic pronouncements even though nobody really understands how the brain works, especially a child's injured brain.

If we had believed him and stopped trying to teach Jesse new things, the neurologist's dire prophecy would have been fulfilled. But the neurologist was right about one thing: Jesse wasn't "intellectually normal." He was intellectually superior. Take that, Doctor God. Of course, I never heard from him again. But I like to think he hesitated before asking parents in code if they planned to get a good one the next time.

Of course, my rage was born of fear, the fear that people like this doctor were right, that I was in denial, that I was putting words in Jesse's mouth. But I knew Jesse was in there. A prophet I met at the Austin airport confirmed it when Jess

was still a toddler (a misnomer because he didn't "toddle" anywhere).

Chris was filming a movie and Jess and I were visiting. As
we waited for Chris to meet us, I saw a frail blond teenage girl
slumped in a wheelchair not far from us, her head down almost
to her chest. She was alone and obviously waiting for someone,
too. She didn't look "intellectually normal." I brought Jesse to
her and introduced him and myself. I told her Jess had cerebral
palsy, not expecting any answer, just wanting to let her know I
acknowledged her. She lifted her head and I was staggered by
the intensity in her deep blue eyes. I think I even took a step
back, blinded by the light she threw. She spoke with a lag in
her voice, the emblematic speech of cerebral palsy that draws
out every syllable, slowing words down, sometimes garbling
them beyond comprehension. But I understood her.

"Can he talk?"

"No, he can only say a word or two," I replied.

"I know how frustrating that must be. I only learned to talk
when I was eight."

Would Jesse learn to talk when he was eight? I didn't know
then that he would never speak in full sentences like this blond
messenger, but I understood that she was telling me to never
give up trying to communicate, that my son was present inside
that little nestling bird body no matter what sounds he was able
to make.

At four, communication got a lot simpler with two signals for
"yes" and "no." Jesse's sound for yes was a kiss sound, a sound
that used to drive me to helpless anger when I lived in New
York City and it followed me everywhere, dripping wetly from

the lips of blubbery sidewalk creeps. From Jesse's lips it was the sound of freedom, of discourse, of choice. He could shorten the kiss sound to a click for emphasis. And his "no," the actual word, gave him a light shaft of power over his powerless body. He had a choice, in as elemental a matter as food. Peanut butter, not mac and cheese for lunch. He had the ability to tell me he was Perseus, not Prometheus, when I read him Greek myths and his imagination soared. The window to his soul creaked open.

When Jesse was seven, he enrolled in a program at Boston College that used a new prototype "eye-gaze" computer. Electrodes were fixed on his face, surrounding his eye muscles, and his eyes moved the cursor. Jesse played a video game for the first time using the device. He beat his dad in an alien-smashing game and giggled in the backseat all the way home, his glee erupting over and over until he could only moan with delight, exhausted, triumphant.

He also proved to us that he could read, as I had long suspected. He was reading a first grade book on the computer titled *Just Grandma and Me*. His eye moved the cursor from word to word. One of the pages said, "We wanted to fly the kite, but the wind was too strong." I asked Jesse, "What word up there describes you?" Very deliberately, he hit the word "strong," over and over. "Strong. Strong. Strong. Strong."

Computers moved Jesse forward from reading into writing. We had decided against using the eye-gaze as Jesse's main computer; it would have been impossible at that time to use it in a classroom. But a regular Mac laptop could be adapted to accommodate Jesse's only volitional movement, a raking grasp. We installed a program called Speaking Dynamically that scanned through the alphabet one letter at a time, speaking it aloud. To choose the letter he wanted, Jesse would pull on a little green alien connected to a switch on the computer. I love that little green alien because it reminds me of the pictures NASA sends into space, people with their hands raised, hoping to make contact, just like Jesse.

At ten, he wrote his first poem, laboriously eked out over a period of weeks. Writing a poem on the computer involved great deliberation as he bunched together a string of letters first, then words, into a form that pleased him both visually and verbally.

Jesse's computer system worked for more than choosing one letter at a time, too. The sound could be turned off when Jesse had to take a pop quiz in class. For example, in a high school Latin test, the word *agricola* would appear, and then the computer would highlight possible definitions: "farmer," "soldier," "horse," waiting for Jesse to pull the alien when he saw the option he wanted.

Jesse's vocabulary on the computer became more complex as he grew older, and even included Italian phrases when we spent a month in Tuscany: *Ho fame* (I'm hungry), *Ho sete* (I'm thirsty), *Come sta?* (How are you?).When meeting new friends, he could find out all about them: "What kind of music do you like? Do you have brothers and sisters?"

Jesse met and became friends with Emmy, the little girl who played Chris's niece in *My House in Umbria* during the time we spent in Tuscany. She wrote a poem about Jesse.

The Meeting

"Hello"
I said nervously.
He made a clicking noise with his tongue.
I guessed that meant, "Hi."
I sat down on a chair, two feet away.
We were alone.
His computer started to talk.
"Do you have any siblings?"
It asked.
"Ummm . . . yes, I have a brother and a sister."
I watched as the letters moved across the screen,
Each word having its own moment in the spotlight,
Reading slowly.
He pulled a little string attached to the computer,
Picking the lucky button.
"What is your favorite food?"
It asked.
"Spaghetti," I answered.
"Jesse, do you want to be friends?"
I asked.
He looked directly at me, with his pure soulful eyes.
He clicked his tongue once again.
I smiled.
I guessed that meant, "Yes."
—*Emmy Clarke, 2005*

■

In middle school Jesse met two of his lifelong best friends, Kyle and Jamie, both brilliant, both quirky, both sharing Jesse's love of music and movies and books.

Kyle played Oregon Trail and Where in the World Is Carmen Sandiego? on the computer with Jess, or they watched *Amadeus* or *Whale Rider* on the DVD player, but mostly they liked to lie on his bed and listen to music. Both were into classic rock, Andrea Bocelli, and show tunes. Sometimes they listened to Jess's favorite, Edgar Allan Poe, on tape.

A beanstalk already more than six feet tall at twelve, Kyle was obsessed with words, rolling them on his tongue like fine wine. "Bizarre. I love that word. *Bee-zarre*," Kyle would say, his reedy voice cracking. Jesse would laugh and make his kiss sound in agreement. They could use the computer to speak, but the technology could be clunky and time-consuming. Often I heard laughter and music from Jesse's room and the hum of Kyle's conversation and Jesse's responses. This kid who loved so many words was Jesse's best friend, able to sustain a friendship with a boy whose words were locked inside.

Jamie started out as Jesse's seventh-grade science class partner, a cute, goofy twelve-year-old who favored wearing flannel pajama bottoms decorated with frogs to school. She asked Jess to the middle school prom and they spent long weekends thereafter floating in the indoor pool we had installed for Jess. Jamie would bring a CD mix she had dubbed especially for Jess (*Jesse's Jammin' #1 Hits*), with eclectic songs ranging from Glen Miller's "In the Mood" to Christina Aguilera's "Dirrty." Her dad was a musician, and she already knew then that music would be her life. They would dim the lights in the pool room, and the music blasted forth. Jess wore his special neck float that allowed him to be free in the water, at eye level with Jamie.

I would invent tasks in the nearby laundry room, trying not to linger intrusively, laughing to myself when I overheard Jamie's monologues on school, teachers, and friends interspersed with Jesse's kiss sounds for "yes." The perfect boyfriend. Jamie's mother told me that Jamie talked about Jess for a month at home before she told her mom that Jess was quadriplegic and nonverbal. Her mother, amazed, asked her how they communicated. "Oh, I know what Jess is saying," Jamie said, with a middle-schooler shrug. "I can see behind his eyes."

■

Goody died in his sleep like Jesse, the night before my surgery to remove the Not-Jesse. A few months before his death he began to rouse from his semi-torpid state and act like his younger, joyful self. At least twice I saw him race to the threshold of Jesse's room, then stop short and wildly wag his tail, greeting the empty air with exuberance. I was absurdly jealous of the dog. He was communicating with Jesse. Wasn't he?

The last thing Jesse said to me was "yes," using his kiss sound. I told him I loved him, and he said "yes." I knew the intonations of that kiss. Sometimes it meant an exuberant "Yeah!" like when he heard Mozart in a fifteenth-century church in Prague and the musicians played his favorite piece. Sometimes it was blissful and sleepy, part of a long drawn-out sigh after a massage. It could be sullen, the teenage equivalent of "Yeah, right!" after I yelled at him for goofing off on his studies and threatened to ban a trip to the mall that weekend. It could even be lascivious, like the time Jesse, then fourteen, turned to his friend Luca after watching the tango number in *Chicago* and let out a loud smack, drunk with pleasure at the sight of all those leggy showgirls.

I read over my journals of the early years and I see that I underscore my doubt again and again about what Jesse really was saying. Even when I clearly heard him say, "I love you," I was afraid it was only my yearning that made it so. But I heard unmistakably that last "yes," the kiss sound in response to my "I love you." We sat in our overstuffed green chair in our usual nighttime place: side by side, my arm around Jesse, who leaned his head against my chest. Jesse's eyelids started to droop, and I kissed him good night, nodding to Chris that Jess was ready to be carried to his bed. Jesse smiled sleepily and gave us his kiss sound. I don't know if Jess knew that he would fly away in the night, if there was even a transition between his best dream to fly and the leaving of his body, but that kiss was a "yes" to it all—Jesse's coda, the finale to a life that was lived like a symphony.

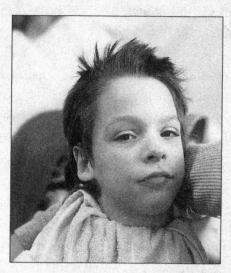

Jesse, age four

QUALITIES: a) funny b) caring c) patient
—*Jesse's Personal Inventory, Health Class, 2003*

CHAPTER FIVE

I'll Be Your Mirror

When Jesse was a baby, the looks he got on the street were mostly of the generic admiring baby-cooing types from the tottering elderlies of Hoboken, the same ones who felt perfectly comfortable telling me to put a hat on him because he looked cold, or to adjust his blanket because he looked hot. When he got older we rolled up towels to keep his lolling head in place in a regular stroller because we couldn't afford fancy adaptive equipment. When it became evident he was disabled, the slackness of his torso muscle tone and the spasticity of his arms and legs elicited different kinds of looks. Some people stared unabashedly, some gave a fleeting look of pity, some looked away quickly as if the mere sight of Jesse would bring a curse down on them.

There were days when the looks didn't bother me and

there were times they sent me whirling back in time to the Lake, the working-class part of Newton, Massachusetts, where I grew up. I stand there, the adolescent mouthy Marianne, hand on hip, face contorted, voice dripping with contempt: *"Take a pickchuh, it lasts longuh, asshole!"* That was then. Now, when people stared at Jesse, I danced a *haka* for them, loudly declaring so the gawkers could hear, "Jesse! You're so handsome, people can't take their eyes off you!"

People looked away, embarrassed at being caught. But it was true. Jesse *was* physically beautiful. He had huge, liquid, saint-like dark brown eyes, and perfectly shaped full lips. A halo of platinum edged his light brown hair and lined his features when he was very young, his inner light made manifest; he had a high forehead and a strong, straight nose, with smooth olive skin that seemed to glow from within. All the features that on my face were too strong looked great on Jess, enhanced by Chris's high brow and curvy lips. The muscle slackness that affected his trunk had spared his facial features. Jesse's face was expressive and mobile, a huge smile often stretching those perfect lips to reveal a row of pearly little baby teeth.

I was so seduced by his beauty I was giddy around him. I wondered sometimes if this was a basic soul flaw on my part. What if he were ugly, a fairy tale monster, a troll? Would I still love him more than my life? Was I shallow? There's a famous photograph by W. Eugene Smith of a Japanese mother bathing her child, hideously deformed by mercury poisoning when corporations released pollutants into the shellfish beds and contaminated the village's water supply in the fifties. The mother, a modern Pietà, looks down at her daughter as she supports her body, floating in a traditional Japanese bathing pool. I recognize that look. She's looking at her child in the same way I looked at Jesse, with helpless, unfiltered love. She sees only a child, her beloved child.

I really wasn't shallow. I was practical. Jesse was going to have a hard enough time in the world. Good looks couldn't hurt. Desmond Tutu said that the worst thing about being singled out on the basis of skin color under apartheid was that it ultimately made a person "doubt he was a child of God." I didn't want Jesse's disability to make him forget that he was a child of God, a member of the human race. And I didn't want him to feel like a freak show for the gaping crowds.

The amazing thing was—this tactic worked. Jesse knew without question he was a child of God. Jesse loved his body, loved the way he looked. He reacted to compliments with smiles of delight. He didn't have fits of depression over the stares, as I would have. I was hyperaware of my looks and whatever was lacking in my appearance because I had chosen a career that judged on looks first, then talent. I was a "character" actor (meaning "not pretty"), which I could live with—it also meant more roles as I got older—but I wanted Jesse to love himself.

Giving Jesse the knowledge of his own beauty worked, because it surrounded him, permeated him, and, most importantly, came from him. My friend John said that Jesse "was the least anxious kid I've ever known" because "though there were parts of Jesse that stayed hidden from us, he had a physical connection, an intimacy with his parents and the other people who cared for him that most people never experience, an intimacy he didn't lose as he grew older." Jesse knew the sensual pleasures of being held, kissed, cuddled, *loved,* far longer than most people.

I was always aware of people looking at us when we were out in the world, and we took Jess everywhere: to fancy restaurants, coffee shops, amusement parks, concerts, plays. Chris and I often felt like the lone family with a disabled kid in all those places. Where were the others? How come we never saw them? Were they all hidden away somewhere? We knew what it felt like to be a minority now. At the park, or some other family outing, we wanted to lock eyes with another family who *knew,* not just the everyday families who gave us sympathetic or curious looks.

Nothing was normal about our family anyway. In the early years, before Jesse started school (and even after that), we lived like nomads, traveling to film sets on different locations all over the country, staying in five-star hotels like royalty, then returning to our working-class Hoboken apartment above a store. Once, in Austin, Texas, we were having dinner in a restaurant. The people in the booth next to us kept turning their heads and staring all during dinner. They were pissing me off. *Rude!* Just as I was about to flip over into Lake mode (*"Take a pickchuh!"*), the guy in the booth addressed Chris: "Hey, weren't you in *Lonesome Dove?* Dayum, that was great!"

Chris had played July Johnson in the Larry McMurtry miniseries *Lonesome Dove* the year before, and that cowboy tale was iconic in the Lone Star State. As Jess got older and Chris did more and more films, the looks and double takes were more often directed at him—although Chris was such a chameleon in his parts, most people thought they might have gone to high school with him, or that they had seen him at the dump or supermarket.

Still, alone with Jesse I was vigilant, feral, a mother grizzly rising to towering monster heights and ready to step in and body-block any stray looks or remarks when we were out in public.

I accosted the poor woman from *People* magazine who came to interview Chris, practically barring the door of our house.

"You're not gonna write some treacly article about the tragedy of our disabled child, are you?"

The woman looked stunned.

"I didn't know you had a disabled child, honestly!"

"So do you promise your readers won't need insulin after they read your article?"

And so forth. The article was great, by the way. No sugar overdose.

Another time, in Montana, our breakfast in a small hotel was interrupted by someone from a nearby table, who came over to us choked with tears.

"I just want you to know that I have never seen such a loving family."

That was nice. We were Ambassadors for Family Love. But there were times we just wanted to be an anonymous family, eating breakfast together. It was true that Jesse generated something ineluctable, a blast furnace of love that sometimes warmed the people around us. This type of declaration happened more often than you would think. I suppose the part that always annoyed me was, did this person think we deserved a medal for loving our "imperfect" child?

I wondered about the people who looked straight through to Jesse, the ones who could actually see him beyond the disability. How did they do that on first glance? The handsome doctor in Tuscany who came to the villa to renew a prescription, smiled at Jesse, and turned to us, declaring, "Jesse *choose* you as parents, you know." The kids in Jesse's elementary school who insisted that Jesse was talking to them. The ones who knew instinctively to address Jesse directly, not speak to me as an interpreter for him.

Before I had Jesse, I would turn away quickly if I saw a severely disabled person on the street or at a store. Assuaging my own fears, I thought that it was probably what they wanted, not to engage. But after Jesse died, I saw him one day in the eyes of a big, unattractive, mentally challenged man at a café where I was having lunch with my friend and Jesse's former tutor, Rachel. He locked eyes with me and I gasped.

Why is Jesse looking at me through that man's body? I looked away, pretended I didn't see him, engaged my friend in distracted conversation while my mind fevered. *Maybe he's trying to tell me that unconditional love comes through different bodies, even big, ugly, mentally challenged men. Maybe I'm losing my mind. Maybe it isn't Jesse shining through that man. I can't tell Rachel. I can't tell anyone. What if my brain just flies away and I start seeing Jesse everywhere?*

So I ignored him. For my own sanity. I ate lunch in the cute little café with my friend and made small talk and didn't look at the big scary ugly mentally challenged man. But when I got up to leave, I sneaked a look at him as I was walking by. He waved, a slight stiff-handed wave, and he smiled, his lip curved in such a familiar way that I froze. My eyes traveled a long, long way, to his. I smiled back and waved.

Hello, Jesse. I see you. You're so handsome, I can't take my eyes off you.

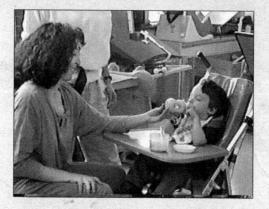

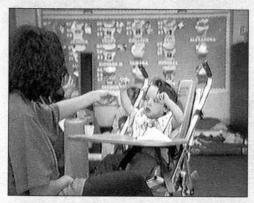

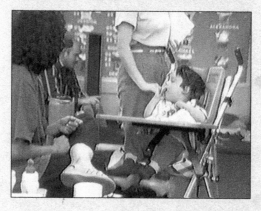

Jesse, age two, at Early Intervention classes

CHAPTER SIX

Early Interference

We were living in Hoboken, the Mile Square City just one PATH train stop away from Greenwich Village. At Elysian Park, just down the street from our apartment, there was a stunning view of the Manhattan skyline, enshrined forever in the film *On the Waterfront*.

On daily walks to the park, when Jesse was still small enough to be stuffed into a Snugli, I would pass a Gothic-looking building that originally housed the Benevolent and Protective Order of Elks. The building looked as if it should be sitting in an empty field surrounded by stunted trees, its gloomy gray brick battered by slashing rain and howling winds, and inhabited only by malevolent spirits. A haunted house on Hoboken's main drag, the BPOE building loomed over Washington Street, its facade dotted with carved elk heads and a life-size gold elk bolted to the sidewalk in front, suitable for worship by pagan idolaters.

Normally, this would be the quirky kind of architecture that would thrill my soul, especially the decapitated carved elk heads, but there was a huge dread-inducing banner draped across the front, advertising an early intervention program for children at risk for developmental disabilities. Under the banner, a sign listed the disabilities the center served. But I was fixated on only one: cerebral palsy. I would walk by the building every day and chant my ward-off spell, which was a fast-pitched *fattura*: "noCPnoCPnoCPnoCPnoCPnoCP."

The spell didn't work. We knew Jess was at risk because of the Grade IV intraventricular hemorrhage he had suffered on the third day of his life. When we went to Children's Hospital in Boston for a second opinion on whether Jesse needed shunts in his brain, we finally got the diagnosis of cerebral palsy with severe spastic quadriplegia.

Cerebral palsy can occur in utero when the baby has a stroke, during birth when the newborn is deprived of oxygen, or after birth because of a cerebral hemorrhage, a distinct danger for premature babies, as in Jesse's case. It is not a genetic disease, nor is it progressive. Once the brain damage occurs, the muscle dysfunction is permanent. We still didn't know what the diagnosis meant for Jesse, though, because he was only seven months old, and "motor control damage" could range in severity, from a slight limp to quadriplegia (all four limbs affected). There could be cognitive damage, too, visual or hearing disorders, seizure disorder, or learning disabilities. We simply would have to wait to see how severe Jesse's condition was. One thing was clear: he wasn't meeting developmental milestones, and could not hold up his head or sit independently.

After Jess was diagnosed, I signed up for the early intervention program in the haunted house on Washington Street. Early intervention programs are government-sponsored classes for children at risk for developmental disabilities from birth to age three. At age three, children transition out of the program, which includes physical and occupational therapies, classes in child care for parents, and social workers who provide assistance in applying for welfare and disability financial support.

Now we needed the services of the early intervention center: on-site physical therapist, speech therapist, occupational therapist, instructor, and social worker. The program was free to all families with at-risk babies and located only six blocks from our apartment. With its help I would put away spells and magical thinking. I would deal with Jesse's condition. I would learn everything I could about how to help my child, and there would be caring professionals to guide me. I cried with relief at the thought of the warm and instructive haven I had found, and the fellowship of other parents of disabled children I would enjoy.

Our first day at early intervention, however, shattered my illusions. The room where the program took place was cavernous, with high ceilings lit by fluorescent lights and acoustics that both raised and muffled normal speech tones. The staff did not seem to know the damage that harsh lights and jangling sounds can do to a baby with an immature central nervous system. On that first day, Jesse was strapped into a reclined seater and placed in a semicircle with the other infants. Parents were seated behind the children and the instructor was in the middle.

The instructor began singing a song naming the infants and parents, and then took the babies through a sequence of banging drums, shaking rattles, and ringing bells. Jesse reacted badly to the lights, noise, and restraints and began screaming and thrashing in his chair. The instructor addressed him firmly, saying, "Jesse, when you stop crying you can come out of the chair." Jesse ignored this unhelpful advice, his screams accelerating to a hysterical pitch. I was told that all the babies reacted this way at first and that Jesse would get used to it. I was not allowed to take him out of the chair and comfort him because "CP kids have to learn independence." Finally, Jesse shut everyone out, his gaze fixed at his side.

I wonder how many "normal" babies are independent at five and a half months, Jesse's true age when corrected to reflect his premature birth.

That night I paced the floor of our apartment above the store, smoking, crying, and feeling helpless. I felt for the first time that we had a disabled child, not a baby who might possibly have a disability, because Jesse was at a place that defined him only by his disability ("CP kids"). None of it seemed right. My mother's instinct was to pull him out of the program. But every book I had read and every professional we had consulted had all stressed the need for early intervention. And every professional had also stressed the pitfalls of the "overprotective" mother and the parent "in denial." So I returned to the haunted house for our next session. Things continued to go downhill.

Our session with the physical therapist was a disaster. She roughly stripped Jesse of his outside clothes, and he began to howl. "Well, I can't work with him if he's going to cry all the time," she said.

Jesse was failing physical therapy. Or was the therapist failing Jesse? To watch your child handled roughly is to have a piece of your soul crumple into ash. But physical therapy was important—wasn't it? At least I made some progress with the instructor during the song-and-banging sessions. I asked the instructor to dim the lights, and convinced her to allow Jesse to come out of the chair at the first signs of becoming hysterical. I would calm him down and return him to the chair as soon as possible.

I was looking forward to sharing information with other parents in the group sessions scheduled at early intervention. The neonatal intensive care unit (NICU) had released Jesse to us at two months old without an operating manual and, in the days before the Internet, I had to rely on what books I could find and a newsletter I subscribed to for parents of children who had had intraventricular hemorrhages. I knew no other parents of disabled children. Some of my friends had babies near Jesse's age, but they were all able-bodied and had no medical issues whatsoever. It was hard to see my friend Nancy's precocious little Bobby flying around the room. I felt that I shouldn't be around pregnant friends, as if I was tainting them somehow, as the living embodiment of their worst fears, all realized in me and my baby.

I hoped to find support within the sorority of mothers at the haunted house, but there existed a language barrier too steep to surmount, and an inflexible schedule that bordered on the absurd. During one session I was informed that it was the day for Parent Group, and I should leave Jesse with the instructors and attend. Noting that the only other parents present were two mothers who didn't speak English, I politely declined, suggesting we use the time to work with Jesse. No, today was the day for Parent Group. So I spent forty-five minutes listening to the social worker explain in fractured Spanish how to get social service benefits to the two women who nodded and smiled to my right and left. I could hear Jesse screaming in the next room through the entire futile lecture.

Released from this fiasco, I arrived back just in time to hear the speech therapist telling my son, "Jesse, when you stop crying, you can—" I interrupted her by reaching over, unstrapping my son from the chair, and taking him in my arms. She glared at me and said, "You'd better start feeding him in a seat. Otherwise, he's going to look like this." She mimed a severely spastic, rigid child, stiff arms and legs jutting out unnaturally. There must have been some orthopedic reason for only feeding Jesse in a chair, but when he was fussy, I found it easier to feed him cradled in my arms, ensuring that he actually ate something.

The next morning I wrestled anxiously with Jesse during breakfast, the image of the rigid child before my eyes like a nightmare vision of the future. He cried, I cried, and no breakfast was eaten that day.

That uneaten meal marked the turning point. I ended the program with the physical therapist at the center and hired a gentle, positive therapist who made home visits. She did not even touch Jesse until near the end of the first session.

We withdrew Jesse from the entire program and bought lots of books. Chris and I learned the proper neurodevelopmental techniques for holding, feeding, and bathing our child. Jesse didn't miss the "stimulation" of being restrained in a chair and having bells and rattles shaken at him. We had lasted a month at the early intervention center in Hoboken.

I wrote an article titled "Early Interference" for the September 1989 issue of *Exceptional Parent*, a magazine devoted to parents of children with disabilities. It caused a furor. The next issue was devoted to a forum where parents and administrators argued the pros and cons of the article. Here's what I said that was so seditious: Parents have the right to determine who deals with their kid, and to choose any educational placement for their kid because, in the end, *it's their kid.* The parents agreed with me; most administrators and professionals expressed the fear that my article would turn parents off from seeking help in the form of early intervention. But I wasn't against early intervention. I wasn't against the organization that ran the early intervention programs, or what they were trying to do. I just wanted to find a place where parents were listened to and Jesse wasn't a "CP kid" first and a kid second.

The resentment that had begun to accumulate in the intensive care unit was now spilling over to the Hoboken early intervention program. Jesse, who had not been our baby for the seven weeks he was in the hospital NICU, was still not our baby. It felt like he belonged to the instructors, therapists, and social workers who were warning us not to be "overprotective."

Chris and I found another early intervention program about twenty minutes away in Hackensack. That one insisted we take part in a "support group" where Chris was always the only man and the social worker leading the group was young and inexperienced. At our intake session, this squeaky-voiced girl asked me solemnly if I "thought I was overprotective of Jesse." Again. Obviously, I was going to have to come up with a stock answer to satisfy the social workers, since this question was on their need-to-know form, apparently right under name, address, and social security number. I toyed with, "Nah. You can keep him if you want."

This social worker ineptly tried to get the mothers "in touch" with their emotions during the support group, an excruciating process that seemed to Chris and me more like prying than helping. We listened to mothers talking about how their husbands wouldn't touch the baby, or how friends had abandoned them, or how their husbands spent all their free time at the Moose Club. We felt blessed that this was not our experience. Our friends were close and supportive, and Chris nuzzled and held Jesse every chance he got. But attendance at this "support group" was mandatory, even though we got nothing out of it, except feeling depressed. The inflexibility of these rules was impossible. On to the next program.

The Millburn early intervention program was about thirty miles away, but it took almost an hour to get there. I drove our secondhand Honda three times a week, navigating the New Jersey highways nervously—I had been living in New York City for seventeen years and hadn't done any driving in that time.

The woman who ran the Millburn program had a grown son with a disability and that made a big difference in the attitude and delivery of services to the parents who brought their children to this program. For the most part the occupational, speech, and physical therapists working there were sensitive and helpful without condescending to the parents or making them feel like they were inept at handling their own babies. I still had problems with the social worker at Millburn, who looked like a pez dispenser in a suit (she had no discernible neck) and treated the mothers as if we had lost serious IQ points in the act of giving birth. All the mothers I knew hated her.

During breaks at the Millburn program, I hung out with a young mother, Sabrina, in the chilly schoolyard. She was only twenty-one years old and had a sorrowful history: three of her brothers were in jail, her sister was on crack, the father of her young son was also incarcerated, and she had another child at home, a four-year-old. She wanted to institutionalize her son, but was talked out of it by her mother, who, according to Sabrina, had a lot to say but "never changes a Pamper—I got the kid twenty-four-seven!" She called me "girlfren" and bitched about the "seditty" social worker—"she as black as I am, girl!" She swung wildly between wanting her disabled son out of her life and picturing the day when she would walk down the street holding his hand, a dream I knew would never come true. I had never met anyone like her. I admired her feisty spirit as much as I wanted to cry for her. I was amazed at the people Jesse brought into my life.

■

Eighteen years later, I watched a video of Jesse being evaluated at the Millburn early intervention center. The new speech therapist stands beside me to observe as I feed Jesse. She is a pretty woman in her early thirties. She watches with interest, her kind features intent on my son. She is there to help, but as always, I have the uncomfortable feeling of being judged.

In the video I am scarily thin, a sleep-deprived woman in her thirties with a gigantic wedge-shaped Cleopatra hairdo. I appear to be dressed in whatever clothes I picked up from the floor that morning and threw on in a hurry. Jesse is around eighteen months old, finally pudgy, with long cowlicky hair and a smirky smile, wearing his Question Authority T-shirt and jeans. He sits in an adapted chair, one that reinforces his trunk so that he can sit up; his head is kept in place by plastic wings on either side. He makes adorable cooing sounds and shrieks, which I mimic slavishly, like someone chanting a religious text. Jesse is gobbling a cookie, and I am thrilled, as though he just vaulted a thirteen-foot hurdle in the Olympic finals. I giggle with delight, watching him chew openmouthed, only dragging myself away from his sunlike presence to look over at the speech therapist to make sure she shares in the wonder of this feat. Look at him chewing! Look how he swallows! I am so in love with him that I look like a cult member. I am also aware that I am the first line of defense for Jesse and, however unreasonably, I want my attitude to be the rules of engagement for dealing with him.

It didn't always work.

Jesse's physical therapist at Millburn could have been the model for the woman in the *American Gothic* painting. She never smiled. She left red finger marks in his arms, and answered his cries while she manhandled him with "Life's tough." I hoped she'd never have to know just how tough life was for Jesse Cooper.

Even now, eighteen years later, while watching the video, I want to reach through the screen and leave a black-and-blue tattoo around that therapist's upper arms, a little memento from Jesse's mother. But if I'm completely honest, I have to admit that the video also shows Jesse smiling up at her. Appeasing his tormenter? I don't think so. I think he honestly liked her, and that is what kept me from replacing her, though I remember hovering exceptionally close during her sessions with him. If Jesse had shown fear or cried at her approach, she would have been gone. I learned to trust Jesse's responses from our first experience with "early interference."

I also learned that parents should become actively involved with their child's stimulation and therapy. The way to encourage this involvement is to impress upon parents that they need to carry over the special techniques used in therapy to the everyday handling and feeding of a child at home.

Professionals need to learn that bullying does not help. Worst-case scenarios and gloomy predictions foster a sense of helplessness that is compounded by anxiety and depression. The parent of an at-risk child is given often-conflicting advice by many different professionals on every aspect of raising that child. If the parent makes a personal choice on an aspect of child care that has nothing to do with that child's health problem, let the parents assume control in that area. Each child is a unique individual, and if professionals cannot see the child instead of the disability, they should not work in programs that involve kids.

When Jesse "graduated" from the early intervention program in June 1990, preparations began immediately for placement in a preschool in the fall. Jesse would be segregated from his able-bodied peers and not included in a regular classroom. For those meetings, I would have to get my own Question Authority T-shirt. I would need to use on-the-job training to negotiate my way through another haunted house, the one where the school administrators and their business-as-usual prejudices lived. The yearslong battle to get Jesse out of the haunted house of segregation and into the mainstream of education was about to begin.

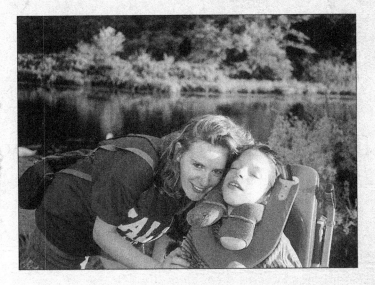

Bernadette and Jesse, age eight, in Plymouth

"Ah! He's himself, he is."

—Bernadette

CHAPTER SEVEN

Blessed Bernadette of Athy

Journal, 1990: *I'm afraid when I look at myself in the mirror, so I avoid it. Some days I spend less time on personal hygiene than a bag lady. My hair is totally gray. Jesse's crying now. It's eleven p.m. and promises to be another long night . . . I remain wearier than I ever thought possible, and yet unable to sleep . . . just let me sleep for eight (or, God, even ten!) hours, please. The impossible dream.*

I was so tired I dreamed of uninterrupted sleep the way a lifer dreams of flying through prison bars. I wanted sleep more than sex, more than food, more than anything I could think of, except for my long list of wishes that involved Jesse, the ones that always began and ended with this: Let him thrive.

Chris was away a lot during Jesse's first and second year, filming a miniseries in Texas and Montana. My family was far from Hoboken—in Boston—and I found myself going to auditions wearing Jesse in a sling like a fashion accessory, or leaving him with my agent while I raced to appointments. On days when I had no auditions, there were early intervention classes, along with doctor's appointments, the myriad chores of a single mother, and what research I could do before the Internet existed—which was precious little.

Bernadette was the first person to answer the ad I had placed in *The Irish Echo*, the New York–based newspaper known to harried parents as the "nanny bible."

She sat in our cluttered dining room, a great cloud of strawberry blond curly hair framing her elfin features, her slight figure barely making a dent in the futon on the loveseat frame Chris had built. She hailed from Athy, not far from Dublin, and had a delightfully low voice, layered with a thick brogue. She told me she wanted to stay in the States and had aspirations to someday become a nurse. Her brother and sister were living in New Jersey, and her parents and one other brother, a priest, were home in Ireland. She lived two blocks from our apartment in Hoboken with her sister, Angela. Bernadette was in her early twenties, but she had an aura of maturity and competence beyond her years. I almost felt like she could parent *me*. I hired her on the spot, without references. I, the Overprotective Mother Extraordinaire, the bane of every medical or therapeutic person who came within three feet of my son, signed Bernadette on after our first interview.

This is why: on seeing Jesse for the first time, Bernadette gasped, "Oh! Isn't he *gorgeous!*"

And her arms reached out for him.

Not "oh, the poor little thing." No look of pity. No edging away, as if disability were contagious. Bernadette spent four hours with Jess on that first day, unable to resist holding him, touching him, cuddling him. Jesse gurgled, smiled, laughed, entranced by that voice, those gentle arms. I was right to follow my instincts. Bernadette stayed with our family for almost five years, becoming a lifelong member of Team Cooper Against the World. She started work the day after Jesse's second birthday, on October 16, 1989. Besides her well-earned vacations, she took only one day off in all that time. She came with us to doctor's appointments, therapy sessions, Jesse's early intervention classes, on movie sets, and on vacations. We visited Montana when Chris was filming and she turned the heads of all the horse wranglers, their eyes following her appreciatively as she pushed Jesse in his stroller past the dappled horses in the corral.

When Chris, I, and even Jesse had parts in John Sayles's film *City of Hope,* Bernadette played an extra in a bar scene and blushed furiously every time she ran into Vincent Spano, the darkly handsome lead and her secret crush. We lived in a hotel in Cincinnati for six weeks while we worked on the film, crossing state lines in frantic doomed searches for green vegetables for Jesse and swimming every day in the indoor pool on the top floor of the hotel.

Our best adventure with Bernadette was in Texas. We were visiting Chris on location in Austin when Mary Kay Place, Chris's costar in the movie, told me about Christ of the Hills, a Russian Orthodox monastery in nearby Blanco that had a portrait of a

Madonna that wept tears of myrrh. A Russian Orthodox monastery in the tumbleweed hills of south Texas? That was weird enough, but the weeping portrait was the clincher—we had to see this. After twelve years as a parochial school prisoner of war, I was into religion only for the art and the kitsch. (My mother had a nonironic Virgin of Fatima lamp and a transgender picture of Jesus that turned into Mary if you wiggled it.) On the other hand, if mystical tears of myrrh could help Jesse, I would let the monk put a magic cotton ball to his little forehead. You never know.

We piled into the rental car and finally arrived after getting lost a few times. The grounds of the monastery were simple, unadorned, but the little chapel was magnificent, filled with gold-tinted icons covering every square inch. The weeping Madonna was kept in another building a few feet from the chapel, and we were led there by a skinny little monk who bore a strong resemblance to Rasputin: long greasy hair, a full straggly beard, and a stained, rusty-looking cassock. Mary Kay whispered that she'd make a donation of dandruff shampoo for the monk's hair affliction.

Bernadette entered first and reverentially stood before the weeping portrait, head bowed. She was religious, and went to Mass on Sundays; her bred-in-the-bone politeness prevented her from comment the numerous times I had gone off on anti-religion rants. The monk took a cotton ball and dabbed her forehead as Bernadette blessed herself. I was next. I stood there, holding a rambunctious Jesse under his arms to face the monk. We waited, holding our collective breaths as the holy moment came. The monk leaned over to daub Jesse's forehead.

There was something spidery about him as he crouched over us. Jess let out a rebel yell and double-kicked the priest where it counted. The monk bent over, hugging his knees, praying, I assume, to the Weeping Madonna to give him back his breathing capabilities. In a supreme act of will, I kept myself from hysterical laughter and we beat it out of there, giggling all the way back to the hotel. Mary Kay never got anointed at all. We raced by the cotton balls stained with the Virgin's tears that were for sale on the way out ($3 a ball).

What Bernadette, Mary Kay, and I didn't know, Jesse somehow did. In 1999, seven years after our visit, the monastery was closed down when it was discovered that child abuse and pedophilia had been going on there for years. Samuel Greene, the founder of the monastery, who was also known as "Father Benedict," and four other monks were put in prison. And the picture dripping holy myrrh? Greene admitted it was a fake. Jesse, as it turned out, didn't need the "holy" myrrh, but he did need Bernadette, who defined holiness in the purity and grace of her service to him.

I watched Bernadette working with Jesse on the mat in our living room, and she was so magnificent I wanted to weep. I would often be distracted by the mere sight of him, so funny and beautiful, lying there marching, marching, his arms swinging and his face set in a determined semi-frown, semi-smile. When Bernadette would hold him upright and he lifted his little legs to walk, it was like viewing something sacred.

One of the reasons I admired Bernadette so much was that she concentrated on what he *could* do, and scrupulously followed instructions from Jesse's various therapists to encourage speech and movement. She was with us through scary seizures and interminable teething, always compassionate, always upbeat. She overcame her natural shyness to march in the Hoboken Halloween parade with us, me dressed as a pregnant nun and Jess as baby Elvis, complete with Velcro sideburns and a red satin cape with a stand-up collar, both created by Chris. The pregnant nun nearly undid Bernadette, but she gamely went with us in and out of the stores on Hoboken's main drag offering candy to kids in costume.

Bernadette had a no-nonsense side that benefited Jesse where sentimentality would have harmed him, holding him back. When I told my mother that Jesse balked at stretching his tight limbs during therapy, she said, "Eh. Maybe no make-a go, then." But Bernadette understood the importance of keeping Jesse's limbs supple, even when he complained, even when it felt like child abuse to me. Why would anyone deliberately take away that heartbreaking smile? But Bernadette persisted, stretching his limbs, positioning him as the therapist directed, making sure his little legs didn't scissor by putting pillows between his knees, patiently opening his tiny closed fists, fitting them around toys. She was strong, stronger than I was in these daily struggles. Jesse's natural beauty and charm would allow him to coast, and I needed him to be a warrior boy for all the future challenges he would face.

Chris and I got to go away on our first weekend alone in two years because Bernadette was the only person on the planet we trusted with our son. We went to a hotel on the Jersey shore and basically slept for two days, sweet untrammeled slumber. We came home to our second-floor Hoboken apartment renewed. A determined Bernadette proudly informed us, "He knows his colors. Show them red, Jesse!" She sat on the therapy mat on our living room floor with Jesse between her legs, supporting his head and back against her chest. Jesse lifted his little fist and hammered down, hitting the red key on his Light 'N Sound piano. Bernadette looked down at him, beaming, proud as any parent.

"Ah! He's himself, he is!"

Bernadette helped Jesse become himself. She helped me to accept help. She never judged my mothering abilities or me. I never felt with Bernadette the accusations I perceived from a lot of people: What did *you* do wrong? How did you get this kid? I often found myself gabbling a litany of innocence to people I had just met, a charm to ward off judgment: I never drank when I was pregnant, never smoked, never did drugs. It wasn't genetic; my gene pool wasn't polluted: it just happened, okay?

Bernadette accepted me, accepted Jesse as he was. I discovered how eager I was to share Jesse with the people who "got" him. To them I offered him up like a poem that explained the cryptic core of love. Chris, of course, was already there, and now Bernadette had joined us. We were blessed. Jesse knew his colors, and he was on his way to knowing himself.

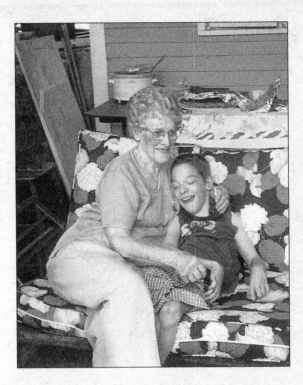

Ma and Jesse, age thirteen, at a family party

"Strega Nona! . . . Teach me your magic, too!"
—*from* Strega Nona's Magic Lessons *by Tomie de Paola*

CHAPTER EIGHT

Things I Learned from My Mother

RELIGIOUS INSTRUCTION

God doesn't require mothers to go to church.

If you leave the bread upside down, God cries.

If you become a nun, you'll wash the priest's underwear for free for the rest of your life.

If you don't wash your face before you go to church, God won't see you.

You can pray to statues of the saints and if they don't give you what you ask for, you can punish them by turning their faces to the wall.

There is no God.

Sexual Instruction

God opens up your stomach to let the baby out when the time is right.

If you wash your hair when you have your period, you'll go mental.

If you swim when you have your period, you'll get sick and die.

If you go into the wine cellar when you have your period, the wine will turn.

If you have sex when you're a teenager, people will be able to tell because you'll suddenly look older.

Not wearing a bra will make your breasts hang to your waist before the age of thirty.

You should dress like a prostitute to look sexy.

The movie *Raging Bull* is a love story.

Men are God.

Men are assholes.

General Instruction

Milk and spaghetti are a poisonous combination.

Too much reading will make you go blind.

Too much reading will make you go crazy.

Too much reading will make you a man.

Too many compliments will bring down a curse on you.

You can be so smart, you're stupid.

Someday your children will make you suffer like you made me suffer.

I did make my mother suffer. We were mortal enemies throughout my adolescent years. She hated the music I played, the ragged jeans and black turtleneck I wore every day. The nonstop reading, which she considered equal to laziness. The sullen face—"that puss," she called it. The smart mouth—*la lingua di vipera*. I would sit in our living room, a stone-cold teenager watching her cry after another screaming fight, ignoring her sobs, suggesting icily, "Why don't you just get back up on the cross where you love to be."

I hated her then. The daily drama. The martyrdom. The simmering resentment. The silent treatment. It was only after I had Jesse and Chris was away for months at a time that I thought of what it must have been like for a forty-three-year-old woman to be widowed with three kids, few marketable skills, and a rudimentary grasp of English.

My mother was a world-class worrier. She spun out sticky threads of worry that brushed my face and enfeebled my limbs when I wanted to do anything she deemed dangerous. She and I would recite the same litany after every one of my declarations:

"I'm stayin' up to watch the late movie."

"You gonna ge' sick!"

"I'm gonna swim out past the raft."

"You gonna ge' sick!"

"I'm goin' to college."

"You gonna ge' sick!"

Oh, it just made my brain explode, her worrying. How could she worry so much about me? She had come to this country alone, at eighteen, a skinny little *contadina* from the mountains of Abruzzi, and was put to work a few days later in the garment district of Boston, before she knew more than a few English phrases. It took courage to do that. But for her children, she was always waiting for the anvil to fall out of the sky. For the wolf to slink down from the mountains behind her house and come through the door of our house on Bridge Street. The worst-case scenario. The *miseria* waiting to happen.

I had decided that the rest of my life would not be lived in fear of what could happen. I wouldn't be like her—I refused to be like her. And then I had Jesse. I worried that he wouldn't survive his first week. Then, when he did survive, I worried that he would be blind, deaf, mentally challenged, unable to walk, unable to talk, unable to feed himself, toilet himself. I worried he would have seizures. And a lot of my worries came true.

And then . . . I stopped worrying.

When Jesse was three, Chris and I took him to a local production of Handel's *Messiah* in Hoboken. He sat in my lap as various soloists sang excerpts. He was alert and quiet during most of the selections, but he came alive during the Hallelujah chorus, squirming in excitement. He began to sing, too. People turned their heads to look, because the event wasn't exactly a sing-along. Instead of being embarrassed, I was thrilled at his little voice striving to join the chorus. In a stop-time moment of joy, Jesse taught me that if I

worried about who was looking at us, or worried that he was be-
having "inappropriately" or maybe—worst-case scenario—about
to have a seizure, I would miss the moment I was in with him, the
moment in time when he was trying to sing the Hallelujah chorus.
And I would miss out on singing it with him. Jesse taught me to
stop waiting for the anvil to fall, or I'd miss the song.

It wasn't an epiphany. The worry only receded to a low-
pitched refrigerator hum. It could still ratchet up to what felt like
a plague of locusts trapped in my head. It was a lesson I had to
learn over and over: Stop waiting for the next crisis. This smile
is for right now. This contentment is now. Jesse was trying to
teach me, but I was a remedial student in the disability parenting course and continued to receive only flashes of knowledge.
Then again, my mother had been my primary school teacher,
and from her I learned the basic alphabet of worry.

My mother's role in our family was High Queen of Drama.
When she wasn't at the climax of a scene, she was building
toward it. When there wasn't even enough material for a scene,
she created one.

After Jesse had arrived ten weeks early, I sat in the tiny
shared hospital room at St. Vincent's in Greenwich Village and
dialed home. I stressed that Jesse was alive and stable, and that
I was okay, but she was so hysterical she couldn't have heard
me. "Buh—it's too soon! Too soon!" she kept yelling over what
I was saying. Ten minutes later, Aunt Ellie called and seemed
shocked that I answered the phone. She was as hysterical as
my mother, but I could just make out the words through her
sobs: "Your mother said you were *dead*!" Dead. How long did
she think she would get away with that one? I realized it didn't

matter; for a Drama Queen it was only about the rush of adrenaline you got in the hysteria of crisis, and it didn't matter if the rush was over in a few minutes when reality set in.

There was no way anyone could call my mother on her drama. Chris and I and Jesse visited her when Jess was a year old. The weekend went fine, but I sniped at Chris the morning we left. He had overslept, and now we would hit traffic driving back to Hoboken. Two days later I got a call from Ellie.

"Ah, Marianne, your mother says you picked on Chris all weekend. She said you're really lettin' yourself go since you had Jesse. He's with all those actresses from Hollywood. She thinks he's gonna leave you if you keep pickin' on him."

I fumed. I had carped at Chris exactly once the entire weekend. Now he was planning to leave me for an "actress from Hollywood," in my mother's soap opera fantasy transmitted via Ellie. Chris found it all highly amusing.

The next time Ma called, I was ready for her. The conversation went like this:

Ma *(standard mournful voice)*: Hi.

Me *(weak, snuffling voice)*: Hi.

Ma *(instantly alert)*: What! Whatsamatter?

Me *(choking)*: Nothing.

Ma *(ramping it up)*: WHAT? WHAT HAPPENED?

The "Nothings" and "Whats?" went on for a while longer. Finally:

Me *(broken up)*: Chris left. I don't know where he is. He's staying with someone in the city.

Ma *(Unintelligible Italian/English hysteria interspersed with shrieking.)*

I let this go on for a while, laughing silently—which sounded like crying to my mother—then handed the phone to Chris.

Chris: No, Ma, but that's what you get for starting this whole—

Ma: SominaBITCH! *(And more in this vein.)*

My sister, Lindy, came home from work to find Ma sitting at the kitchen table with a glass of blackberry brandy. She normally never even had wine with dinner.

Ma: You sister's makin' me DRINK!

Two months later, we visited again, for Christmas. Lindy had videotaped my little niece Jennifer's preschool Christmas show while Chris and I and Jesse did some shopping. My mother had provided a running commentary during the taping, unaware she was being recorded. She prepared me for it, as we were about to view the video.

"Uh, Marianne, I said some things. . . . "

And there it was: her mournful voice-over droning in the background of Jennifer's pageant, like some *strega* chanting an arcane spell.

Ma *(deep sigh):* I dunno, Leendy. I'm worried about Marianne. She's really lettin' herself go. . . . Chris is gonna leave. . . .

It's ironic that I chose acting for a career, given how my mother's never-ending drama exasperated me. But I tried to restrict the expression of my inherited Drama Queen gene to the stage. I've never gotten to play a character like my mother, but still she has colored every one of my roles in some way. I once asked my mother if there was theater in the village where she was raised. She told me there were traveling operas and the Running Madonna.

What was my mother like with Jesse? His birth was the Mt.

Everest of worry, the blood-sacrifice heart of drama. And Ma's first meeting with him wasn't promising. He was still in the neonatal intensive care unit. My mother, Ellie, and Lindy came to New York for a visit. Ellie and Lindy cooed at him lying in his little plastic coffin. Now four weeks old, he was no longer hooked up to various snaky electrodes. My sister held him. My mother, overcome, made a hasty sign of the cross over him and turned away, terrified by all the bleeping machines, the gliding nurse overseers, the Lucite barriers to touching, smelling, holding her grandson.

She felt the blasphemy of this place, as I did, and it aroused in her a primitive, atavistic fear. She hovered fearfully, like an early primate cowering before an eclipse. It was strange to see her so timid, especially in the presence of a baby; child care was an area where she normally had the upper hand. She was no match, however, for this brave new world laboratory of wizened little preemies. Fat equals healthy to someone who grew up where food was not plentiful, and Jesse was not an ordinary, fat, kicking newborn. My mother would not be able to teach me basic mothering skills. Instead I would instruct her.

Worry can be unlearned. Its coils can be unspooled from the brain no matter how deeply they're embedded, just as someone can pull up roots and leave their country, their family, friends, and home. Ma braked her worry impulse, because our roles had been reversed. Now she followed my rules: no worrying, no hesitating, no walking on eggshells around my boy. She learned from me how to hold him, spastic legs separated by her knee when he was facing front. She learned from me how to feed him—depressing the spoon lightly on his tongue to prevent thrusting. I know now that her love for me was stronger than her most basic worry impulse, and that deep love spurred her to overcome it. It took me a long time to figure this out, but then again, like she said, you can be so smart, you're stupid.

I didn't have to teach my mother to love Jesse. She loved him, though she was shy with him when he emerged out of baby-hood. She was shy with all her grandchildren when they became kids with distinct personalities, personalities that had to fight for selfhood against her own dominant temperament. When she began to understand Jesse, when she could trust his responses, she lost her shyness. His powerful personality complemented hers. She sought him out at family parties, and there are pictures of her sitting with him when he got older, her arm around him, the two of them smiling complicitly. She enjoyed lying beside him on his bed listening to Italian folk tales on tape and pushing his wheelchair around the mall. She fed him her special pasta and to-die-for *pizzelle* and anise cookies. I even took her to watch him windsurfing, and that was her hardest test. She paced the beach, her eyes on the tiny speck of a sail in the distance, gnawing her hand, holding back tiny shrieks. Jesse's inability to speak made her closer to him; her own grasp of English remained tenuous even after sixty years in this country. She whispered secrets to him that none of the rest of us ever were privileged to hear.

Ma remained a Drama Queen until the end. Jesse enjoyed her rants on subjects from Bill Clinton ("What he do wrong? He had sex! So what?") to his own mother ("Looka you mother, Jesse. Walk around, smoke, talk, act crazy! Whadda we gonna do with her, huh?"). Jesse would laugh appreciatively and lurch his arms toward her, trying for a hug. He loved her high-energy performances. To him, she was the best show in town.

Ma and I declared a truce after Jesse's birth, and I became able to laugh at the foibles that used to drive me insane. But after the truce there was still one area where she and I were at odds. In her view, Jesse's birth had canonized me as La Madonna Sanctissima. But the halo was too tight and gave me a permanent headache. She kept telling me in an awed voice what a great mother I was. I would point out that I got frustrated like everyone else, that I lost my temper and yelled like everyone else, and that I didn't always make the best choices for my kid. "No," she would tell me in a reverential almost-whisper, "you a good mother, Marianne. The best."

Hearing this always inspired dread. Wasn't she the one who warned me about too many compliments bringing a curse down on me? And it made me feel both lonely and sad. Lonely, because in the rarefied regions of sanctified motherhood, the air was thin and no one else was around. Sad, because she was telling me she didn't think if she were in my position, she would be able to do for me what I did for Jesse. I didn't believe that. Case in point: when I was in the tenth grade, shortly after my father died, I committed some heinous crime like talking in class. The nun in charge kept me after school and told me I had been "running wild" since my father died. I was crushed. I told my mother. She and Aunt Ellie swooped down on the unfortunate nun like avenging angels and left her clawed and bleeding. And this was just for getting me upset. Why did she not think she would do even more if I had been as helpless as Jesse? Sometimes, she was so smart she was stupid.

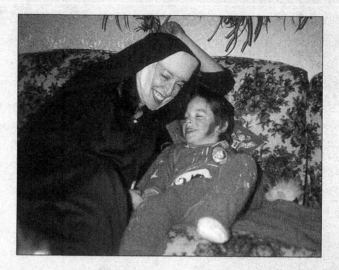

With Jesse, age three, at a Halloween party

The most important lesson I can teach
is to see people for what they can do
and not for what they cannot do.
—*Jesse's autobiography, sixth grade*

CHAPTER NINE

Heretic

The root meaning of the word *heretic* is "able to choose," a fun fact I thought about a lot in 2002 when we stayed at the Hotel Ponte Sisto in Rome. We were a stone's throw from the Campo de' Fiori, where Giordano Bruno was burned at the stake in 1600 for believing in reincarnation and the possibility of life on other worlds. He was a heretic because he was able to choose his beliefs. I am, too. I am able to choose. Bring on the auto-da-fé and light my fire.

Thirteen-year-old Jesse, Chris, and I sat at a wrought-iron table on a sun-drenched terrace, eating breakfast at the Ponte Sisto. We were surrounded by a group of Irish tourists, and their lilting voices, soft as mourning doves' coos, fluttered all around us. I stepped over to the bar for a cigarette while Chris stayed at the table with Jesse. An older man with a gravelly

Dublin accent engaged me in conversation. I asked him if he'd been to the Vatican and seen the artistic wonders there.

"Ah, y'know dese churches were built by nuttin' but slaves. Sure, all of them cardinals was rich and usin' the poor for slave labor. That's how them churches got built. Slave labor."

I murmured that there did seem to be a disparity between the great wealth of the church and the poverty of most of her followers. The man grunted an assent, satisfied. He looked over at Jess and lowered his voice.

"Will ye be takin' the lad to Lourdes, then?"

This guy pretty much summed up my seesaw sense of religion.

I had been raised up in a religion based on fear, subjugation, humiliation, and lurid images of torture and martyrdom. My first exposure to the idea of God was conveyed to me via the Sisters of St. Joseph in kindergarten at Our Lady Help of Christians School (I guess Muslims and Jews could forget about any help from this Our Lady). At four years old, I wasn't sure if my teachers were men or women, or even if they belonged to the human race. I still believed in fairy tales, Hansel and Gretel, Sleeping Beauty, gnomes, sprites, trolls, and all measure of fantastical creatures, both malevolent and benign. The nuns didn't look like any humans I had yet encountered in my short life.

They wore long black gender-masking gowns and white overstarched wimples that tightly framed their fleshy, chapped faces. What they most resembled was the über-evil Wicked Witch of the West from *The Wizard of Oz,* except the nuns' faces were red, not green. I understood that they were as powerful as the Wicked Witch, especially when they meted out punishments and delineated the rules of their strange alternative universe. Instead of hurling a fireball, the nun could lock you in the coat closet for an indefinite amount of time—or forever to a four-year-old—for breaking the rule about staying in your seat. They could rap your tiny knuckles for missing a note when you practiced piano. And in soft, breathy, excited voices, the nuns described the million different ways you could be tortured, like the martyrs, just for belonging to their religion.

Sister Juventius spun her gory tales as she stood under a crucifix that hung on the classroom wall. On the cross was a dying man with a crown of thorns, blood dripping from his head and a wound in his side, and nails driven through his hands and feet. He terrified me. And somehow, the tortured man hanging there was our fault, because we were all born with a black stain on our souls called original sin, according to the sister.

Oh, and it was more women's fault than men, because women started it all in the Garden of Eden by eating an apple and disobeying God. So girls were worse than boys, and that's why they couldn't be priests and say the magic words that changed water into wine and bread into the body of Christ that we would eat once we were seven and received First Holy Communion. If we missed Mass even once we would burn in hell for all eternity. In fact, we should be thinking of that—burning in hell—all the time. I developed facial tics and nightmares pondering the martyrs and their gruesome deaths.

Why on earth would I want to pass this child-abuse religion on to Jesse?

Well, for one thing, there were the miracles, as the Dubliner pointed out. I liked the idea of miracles and magic. When

I was a kid I liked the heavy brocade vestments the priests wore at Sunday Mass, which to me were the sine qua non of playing dress-up, the swinging censers that emitted holy perfumed smoke, the statues of the saints with red votive candles in front of them. You could make a wish and light the candles with a long wooden taper for a dime, a bargain because the wish came along with the thrill of handling fire. I liked the May processions where you got to dress like a mini-bride and wear your Holy Communion dress one more time to crown the statue of the Virgin with a circlet of flowers. Most of all, I liked the faraway portraits of the saints lining the blue ceiling of the church, which I stared at to pass the time during Mass, a mostly incomprehensible ordeal that seemed to last forever.

I liked the package religion came in. It is like a beautifully wrapped birthday present, handed to you by your least-favorite aunt, the impossibly stern one. You remove the exquisite wrapping slowly, regretfully, because what's inside the package can't possibly be as good as the wrapping. And you're right. It's a pair of scratchy gray wool socks that itch when you put them on, mortifying your flesh—a nun-approved present. Your mother gives you a look and you say thank you, but you don't mean it: the socks are disappointing and ugly. You were better off admiring the package than looking inside it.

My parents were a bridge between the nuns' alternate universe. My mother slyly co-opted the church by transforming their rituals into her own folk magic. She had an entourage of saint statues on her dresser, and punished them regularly by turning their faces to the wall if they failed to deliver on a lottery number that had appeared in her dreams. When I was four and the Doberman next door almost took my eye out, St. Francis spent a month facing the wall; he was the patron saint of animals and clearly wasn't doing his job. Ma didn't keep a font of holy water nearby for making the sign of the cross in the nun-approved way. Instead she sprinkled salt into a little bowl of water and dripped oil over it, whispering a secret chant, moving her left hand three times in a circle to ward off the *malocchio* (evil eye). When I was eighteen, she taught me the chant at midnight on Christmas Eve, so she wouldn't lose her own power, she explained.

She didn't regard baptism as a sacrament; it was a spell to protect infants from death. We didn't have a church baptism for Jesse, but to this day I suspect she "baptized" him secretly when she was alone with him. And she performed the evil eye spell many times for him, because, as she warned me, he was a beautiful baby and "Americans," ignorant of the jealous power of the gods, would praise him without adding the automatic anti-*malocchio* phrase "God bless him." The nuns were alien to her, women who rejected men to be married to a ghost, and priests were just men who thought they were better than all of us—at home in Italy, they demanded a dozen eggs to read a letter from America.

My father never went to church, except on Easter and Christmas, to hear the music. The only thing he did religiously was play golf every Sunday. He had abandoned the confessional booth in a rage before I was born when the priest dared to ask him about birth control. "Tell the priests to go work pick and shovel like your grandfather did, they want a baby every year."

How did I end up at Our Lady Help of Christians School

with parents who were basically pagans? They were also immigrants and believed if you paid for something, it must be better. Public schools were free; therefore they weren't as good as parochial schools, according to them and their circle of friends.

It was my father who taught me to question what the nuns were teaching me. I see him standing in front of the bathroom mirror in his shorts, shaving, after a rousing rendition of "Mattinata," the Neapolitan folk song that he belted out every morning to greet the day.

L'aurora di bianco vestita
Già l'uscio dischiude al gran sol . . .
(Dawn, dressed in white
already opens the door to broad daylight)

I stand in the doorway, seven years old, trying to impress him by parroting back the phrases I memorized from the catechism.

"Listen, Daddy. Listen what I learned in school. Who made you? God made me. Why did God make you? God made me to know, love, and serve him in this world and be happy with him in the next."

My father pauses in his shaving and peers down at me, his handsome face masked with soap. I squirm like a puppy in the sunlight of his full attention.

"Why can't you be happy in this world? Somethin' wrong with that?"

I bolted from the church when my father died. I was fifteen, and the nitpicky accountant-like church ruling that sentenced my dad to burning in hell because he missed Mass on Sunday infuriated me. My father, who picked up homeless men from the street, installed them in our rec room in the basement, gave them clothes and food, and put them on their feet. My dad, who raided our closets to send clothes and money to the Old Country for years after the war. My father, this generous man who understood *caritas,* charity, in his very soul was in for an eternity of torment because he golfed on Sunday. None of it made sense. Nor was it right. A tiny idea about injustice was planted.

Ma taught me to appreciate the magic and Daddy taught me to question the subjugation and enabled me to choose for myself what I believed.

We wanted Jesse to know about the world's religions. Chris did not have the primal fear associated with organized religion that still clamped my soul, even as an adult. His exposure had been to Bible verses and sporadic attendance at midwestern Protestant churches that seemed to me as innocuous as a group of Rotary Club members discussing the power of positive thinking. His mother called and asked me if we took Jesse to church. I told her we went every single day, and that our church was a huge rock in the woods overlooking the sea. It was easy to sense God there, and it is where Jesse's ashes now rest, in the soft loam beside the rock.

We read Greek myths to Jesse, along with Bible stories, *The Mountains of Tibet*—a children's book on reincarnation—the speeches of Martin Luther King, the sacred poetry of Rumi and Khalil Gibran. We told him that the basis of every religion was the same: to love your neighbor as you love yourself—which was also the hardest principle to live by. But, in all honesty, to behold Jesse, to see the light shining forth from his helpless body, was to understand that not only was he a pure soul, in that he was incapable of causing others harm, but also to know that his helplessness gave him his greatest power—the power to teach others by drawing out the best in them and, in my case, to recognize that to fight for social justice is to really love your neighbor as yourself.

I am able to choose, and I choose the package: miracles, magic, and art. I choose to reject the teachers of fear and humiliation. I chose Jesse, the one who came wrapped in a beautiful package, and when I looked inside, there was no disappointment; instead I found a teacher of unconditional love, the one truth embedded in every religion.

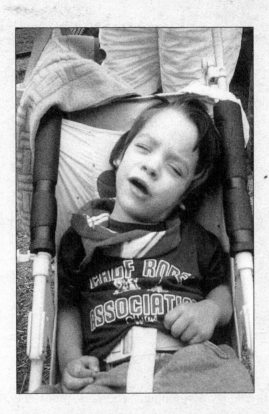

Jesse, age three, in his jerry-rigged stroller

CHAPTER TEN

"Children Like That"

When the heart weeps for what is lost,
the spirit laughs for what it has found.
—*Sufi aphorism*

Heartbreak is incremental when the tally sheet of goals not met belongs to your child. Jesse had met very few physical milestones and could not crawl, walk, talk, sit independently, hold his head up, or grasp objects. We kept moving the goalposts of hope—it's not like we woke up one morning and realized Jesse would never walk or talk intelligibly.

I had a wish list that kept changing:

I wished he would call me "Mommy."

I wished he could hug me.

I wished he could kiss me.

I wished he could look at me head on and smile.

It had become clear that Jesse's physical limitations would be severe. He had no independent physical skills. I watched his frustration when he tried to bring a cookie to his mouth and his arm flailed in the opposite direction, and, mentally mirroring his physical struggle, I had to fight with myself not to automatically do it for him. I knew my interference only mitigated my own pain in each skirmish of the war to control his body. It would not help him. I remember going to my friend Nancy's house and watching her scatter Cheerios on her son's high-chair tray and walk away. Bobby, a few months older than Jesse, reached for the little pieces of cereal with a pincer grasp Jesse didn't have. That glimpse into the world of normality made me feel like a visitor from another planet.

We didn't live in Nancy and Bobby's world. On our planet, I walked the tightrope of sensing when to do things for Jesse and when to let him try something on his own. He would get so frustrated at not being able to crawl that he would bite his own hand and leave marks. We had a "bitey boy" for Jesse to get out his aggravations—an egg-shaped rubber man whose eyes and nose popped out when you squeezed him. I held the egg-shaped man and Jesse sank his teeth into him and latched on. I yelled like a rabid fan on the sideline, "Get him, Jess! Get Bitey!" and Jesse bit with the ferocity of a tiger killing prey.

Bitey never failed to break the tension; Jesse would begin to laugh with Bitey's nose still in his mouth. In a few minutes, he was ready to take on his next physical challenge. If I lifted his chest and crab-walked over Jesse, he could actually crawl around the room, which relieved some of his irritation. He also liked me to "walk" him around the room, with me bent over at the waist and holding him under his arms while he stiffly lifted his little legs, marching in an exaggerated toe-stepping prance. The other tension-breaker was Jesse's swing. Even though he couldn't whirl around the room like a normal three-year-old, he still craved speed and motion. Chris constructed a swing out of a volleyball net and Jesse's adapted soft plastic seat in the doorway between the kitchen and dining room of our Hoboken apartment. I pushed Jess while I cooked dinner, between draining pasta and tossing the salad, and we sang along to the Beatles or Sweet Honey in the Rock. We could reverse the seat to face the dining room so that Jess could keep swinging while Chris and I ate. Listening to music while rocking in the swing was, for Jesse, a daily pocket of bliss.

In the midst of all these changing goals, I realized that Jesse's intellect functioned perfectly, and that is where we centered all our hopes and dreams for him. At the early intervention center in Millburn, Jesse had his first exposure to working on an adapted computer. He made the connection immediately: touch the switch and something happens on the screen. We adapted our computer at home and began using preschool software as a teaching device. We started with Stickybear, a program that displayed simple concepts—above, below, in, out—using cartoon graphics and sound. We couldn't prove that he was reading until four years later, but when he was three he was the enthusiastic recipient of all the learning we could bring to him. The key was bringing the opportunity to learn to him;

his physical limitations made it impossible for him to explore on his own.

The thrill of Jesse's learning was reciprocal, a shared delight. I had been the type of kid who often sneaked away from my playmates to hide in a corner and read. I lived in my imagination as a child, and I wanted Jesse to be able to live in his. The way his face lit up when he learned something new told me that his inner world could transform into an ever-expanding universe, without limits.

At that time I read everything I could by and about disabled writers. I hoped if Jesse had bodily limitations that he could live in his mind like Christopher Nolan, who wrote *Under the Eye of the Clock,* or even produce art like Christy Brown, who wrote *My Left Foot.*

But the limitless universe I was envisioning for Jesse had a black hole in it: convincing others that Jesse's intellect functioned perfectly, and that he was worth educating. The next hurdle would be bringing the learning to Jesse not just at home but in a public school, alongside his able-bodied peers. This would require the school's adapting the curriculum to Jesse's specific learning needs. The name for this is *inclusion,* and it is the holy grail of special education, the object of a quest I didn't yet know I was on.

As Jesse neared the age of three, we began meeting with the Hoboken child study team to discuss his placement for the coming school year. That experience made me consider getting a Bitey Boy for myself. I worried that the "team" would recommend that we institutionalize Jesse, that they would be implacable, that it would become a demand. But I told myself that Bernadette could act as his one-on-one aide and facilitate feeding, toileting, and manipulating objects to help him learn the alphabet and numbers in a regular preschool.

The sheer bureaucratic obtuseness of the parade of bozos that had permanently entered our lives was the worst aspect of Jesse's handicaps. We were treated like overprotective parents for wanting Jesse to participate instead of being strapped into a floor seat and left alone while the more mobile kids banged drums or finger-painted. The no-neck social worker from Millburn clucked about Jesse having Bernadette as his aide, even though the school had no one-on-one aides and Jesse had no independent skills.

The first proposal of the child study team was that we send Jesse to a segregated preschool an hour away, a preschool on the same site as the early intervention program in Millburn. The idea of putting our helpless three-year-old on a bus for a two-hour roundtrip to preschool, even with Bernadette accompanying him, was unacceptable. I didn't want Jesse on a bus for two hours each day. Nor did I want him in a segregated class with no able-bodied kids at all and no chance to hear normally developing language and interact with peers of all abilities. I wanted Jesse to go to preschool in Hoboken, like any other kid.

I was outraged, but the word *overprotective* was being scattershot at me by the bureaucrats in charge, the two social workers, and a psychologist. I was beginning to sense that parents of "damaged" children were expected to hand their children over without question *because* they were damaged.

Paranoid. I was becoming paranoid. Or not. Maybe I was in denial, overprotective. Or maybe I should just follow my own instincts and refuse to hand over my kid. He was helpless.

Would parents of "normal" children allow them to be bused to and from school for two hours every day? We allowed the bus trip for an excruciating week, a sop to the "overprotective" crowd. Jesse was so regularly carsick I was afraid Bernadette would quit. He slept at preschool, exhausted after being sick. We decided to find a preschool in Hoboken.

There was no public preschool in Hoboken in 1990. And in the surrounding area, no public preschools integrated special-needs students with able-bodied students. This meant we had to find a private preschool that would accept Jesse, with Bernadette accompanying him and seeing to his physical needs during school. There was a Catholic school just two blocks from our apartment. Putting my own abusive kindergarten experience out of my mind, I reasoned that things had changed in the thirty-odd years since I had undergone the tyranny of the nuns at Our Lady Help of Christians. And Bernadette would be with Jesse every minute of his time in preschool, which was probably taught by a layperson, not one of the fantastical creatures from my own childhood.

So I called the priest and laid out my case: Yes, Jesse was severely disabled, but he had a personal aide who would see to his every physical need. We wanted him to be around other kids and interact as best he could, facilitated by Bernadette. We wanted him to go to school in his own neighborhood. The priest heard me out, then delivered his verdict.

"You can talk to the sister in charge, but I think you'll find that public school is the place for *children like that.*"

I stammered a reply.

"There isn't. There isn't a public preschool in Hoboken."

I pictured him sitting in his office. Well fed. Looking forward to his dinner, cooked by someone else.

"I went to parochial school for twelve years, you know."

This sounded pathetic even to me. There was a pause. Did I detect a sigh in his voice?

"Well, you can talk to the sister in charge, as I said. But I think she'll tell you what I told you."

The priest hung up. So much for the halt and the lame being welcomed by the parochial preschool in Hoboken.

"Children like that." Why did this remark have the power to lay me low? Why did I still expect kindness and mercy from "religious" figures? I was outraged, but mostly at myself, for being so naïve. Looking back, though, kindness would have undone me. The priest's indifference strengthened my growing resolve to find Jesse a neighborhood preschool. Throughout the struggle there was Jesse, my antidote. Looking at him in his little seater/ rocker, I received his light like a miracle drug that broke a consuming fever. I went back to cold-calling preschools.

We found a secular preschool in a church basement on Washington Street, three blocks away from our apartment. It was gloomy, loud, and crowded, but at least it wasn't two hours away, and the teachers were kind. A physical therapist came twice a week to our apartment, at our expense. We had no occupational therapist, but Chris and I and Bernadette were integrating play with occupational therapy, encouraging Jesse's fine motor skills with puzzles and pegs and computer switches. I attended a workshop that taught me to adapt toys for Jesse so that he could use his little fist to hammer a switch attached to a toy and get a response. Chris glued oversized knobs to puzzles; I spent hours poring over "special needs" catalogs of adapted toys and equipment. One thing was clear: anything for sale in a "special needs" catalog cost easily three times the price of a toy for normal kids, as did adapted sippy cups and Rube Goldberg–looking crazily curved spoons that attached to Jesse's wrist with Velcro but did nothing to tame his wavering arm.

Everything in our little parallel universe was jerry-rigged. I wandered the aisles of toy stores, wondering how I could get Jesse to participate in a meaningful way. Board games with pop-up dice were within his grasp; his little closed fist could pummel the plastic bubble. Adapted video games weren't available until years later. Chris's skills as a carpenter and designer were invaluable. He created a plastic cover that covered the keys of one of Jesse's first computers, leaving only the space bar free for him to hit with his fist. The same went for strollers; Chris covered the bars on either side of the stroller with foam pipe insulation so Jesse wouldn't hit his head during a seizure episode or by spastically jerking his head.

We were trying to cover all the therapies we were missing by not sending Jesse away to Millburn every day. Millburn would have offered physical and occupational therapy, including augmentative technology. We were paying for all of those ourselves, but Chris and I were worried about money. We were always worried about money—acting isn't a profession where you draw a paycheck every week, unless you're on a series or working on the soaps, and even then your character can be killed off—along with your income.

Health insurance was available only if you worked on Screen Actors Guild jobs, and only if you made a certain amount of money within the year. You could pay into the system, but we could never afford it. None of this was important when we lived in our sixth-floor walk-up in Hell's Kitchen, where the rent was three hundred dollars a month. We were healthy twentysomethings, and walked, biked, or took the subway everywhere. We saw free theater when we got tickets at our union, Actors' Equity, and spent any money we had on acting classes, résumé pictures, and a minimal amount of food.

We had no insurance when Jesse was born ten weeks early, and by the time he had spent ten weeks in the NICU, our hospital bill was approaching seventy thousand dollars. It might as well have been seventy million. We had too many other things to worry about besides the hospital bill, like keeping Jesse alive and getting him home to us. I asked Chris, "What are they gonna do, keep him?" In the nick of time, Chris got a job on *The Equalizer,* a weekly television series, and our insurance kicked in to cover the astronomical NICU bill.

Chris got fairly steady work after Jesse came home from the hospital, but getting the insurance to cover Jesse's various needs for doctors and equipment proved to be as tricky as navigating the rocky shoals of what the Individuals with Disabilities Act of 1975 supposedly guaranteed: "a free and appropriate public education." We "had" both, but only on paper. The reality was much more elusive. From now on, we would be fighting a two-pronged battle for both Jesse's inner and outer worlds.

One balmy late-spring evening, I sat with Jesse on our secondhand brown velour sofa. The windows were wide open and we heard the shouts of the wiseguy kids on the corner playing the one-up insult game. I enjoyed the feel of Jesse's little body nestled in my lap. He wasn't stiff tonight; his fluctuating muscle tone was under control. "FUCK YOUUUUU!" echoed from the street, followed by a jackass bray of adolescent laughter. I inhaled Jesse's singular scent, my motherdrug high, better by miles than anything illegally sampled in my misspent youth.

We both stared at the board with magnetic letters propped up on my knees. His preschool was teaching the letters of the alphabet that week. I asked him the first letter of his name. His concentration had the focus of a baby Zen master. I asked him again. His fist slammed the letter *J*, scattering all the other letters onto the floor. I bent to look at him, to drink in the symmetry of his profile. He glowed. He crowed his triumph, *"Uh . . . UH"*— the second "uh" an operatic high C of utter joy. His joy was mine, and I sang his aria back to him: "Uh . . . UH!"

I was overprotective, in denial, and ready to morph into whatever murderous mother-deity I needed to become.

He will learn. He will go to school. Of this I am certain.

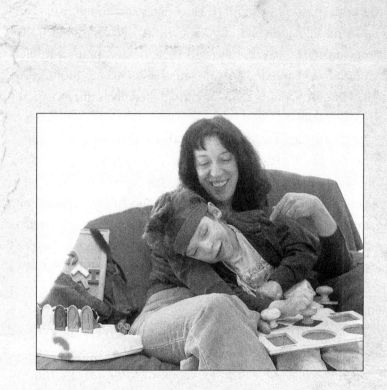

Jesse, age five, with his adapted shapes puzzle

"Oct . . . eight!"

CHAPTER ELEVEN

Incantation

I am hacking at the reeds again today, which is what I do on the days I can't conjure Jesse for this book. I have been trying to call Jesse back to a place where he's alive and five years old and eager to learn about the world around him, but instead I keep finding him dead in his bed. So I stand in the thicket of the parasitic reeds that are taking over the tidal marsh behind my house and I hack at them ineffectually with a giant pincer tool. I extend the pincers straight out to cut the reeds down, making my forearms feel as big as Popeye's after only a few minutes.

I am drawn to the reeds like a sleepwalker, still wearing my pajamas, unprotected from the stinging vines that sometimes curl around the reeds. I don't notice the cuts and scratches on my ankles. Time recedes and there is only the curtain of reeds before me, impenetrable, like a veil. There is a river beyond the veil, a salt river that flows from the sea. I need to break through to the green water that moves in and out of its muddy bed twice a day, as if the Jones River will somehow become the River Styx that carries me to Jesse.

The reeds tower over me, ten feet tall. They sway mockingly as I cut them once, twice, three times, until they are only two feet high. Then I stomp their stems down, the most satisfying and rewarding part of this ritual. When I look up again after stomping, I still can't see the river, and the towering reeds seem to have multiplied, the poofy little quiffs at their very tips doing an obnoxious victory dance in the wind. Their roots spread out like a grid and they're impossible to just yank out. I have an absurd commitment to keep cutting them back and stomping them down. They will come back, because their roots are in the marsh, deep beneath the surface, intertwined like the neuronal pathways of a human brain.

They have a really ugly botanical name, *phragmites,* pronounced "frag mighties." Well, I'm here to tell them they're not that mighty. I'm here to frag them. This is the warrior queen mode I am in today. I turn around, panting, after a particularly enjoyable stomping session, and I see a nesting bird. An ordinary sparrow. In the middle of the crushed reeds I stomped just yesterday, it sits calmly only a few feet away, a strange thing of majesty. I gasp at being so close to a still, wild thing, and fade into the reeds, careful not to frighten it. Then I look closer. It isn't sleeping. The bird is dead. Its eyes are closed and its little brown body looks cozy atop the broken reeds. I say aloud, "Oh. You're dead," as if explaining its condition to the bird.

I am reminded of myself at six years old, the time I found a lifeless baby bird on the ground by the apple tree that scratched its bony branches against my window and kept me up at night fearing apparitions of saints or ghosts. I took the baby bird in my cupped hands and carefully laid its naked body beside the furnace in our cellar, hoping the warmth would revive it. But it never woke up. That was a lesson: Dead is dead.

Finding the bird is the long way to come back to Jesse. Trying to summon him, I was hurled into that moment when his stillness signaled an end and not sleep. He looked comfortable, too, that terrible morning, and his eyes were closed on his bed that had become a bier. But that memory is not where I was headed this morning. That's not where I was planning to go. I don't need to be reminded that Jesse is dead, or that on the day preceding the night he died a bird slammed into the sliding glass door a few feet from where he sat. I don't need to be reminded of my own superstitious dread. It's all there, beneath the surface, like the roots of the phragmites.

I have to keep going, to see if I can summon another place, another time, when he was alive. I turn my back on the bird and hack again at the reeds, cutting them down to raise Jesse up.

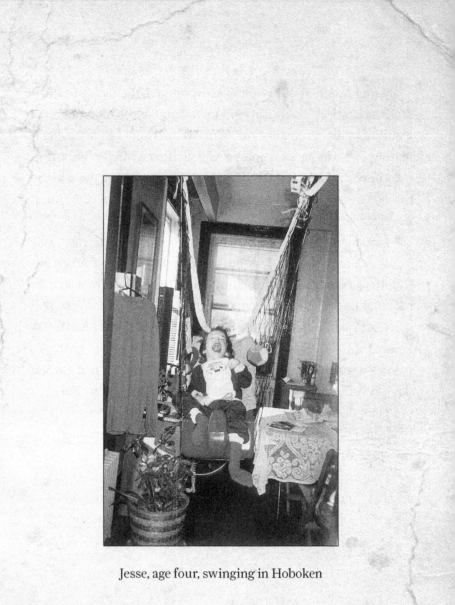

Jesse, age four, swinging in Hoboken

CHAPTER TWELVE

I Am the "Other Element"

In good form at school. Paid a lot of attention, said "Go
home" to Miss Eleanor [speech therapist].
—*Bernadette's kindergarten notes*

Our fortunes had improved and I loved our new apartment
in Hoboken. We had moved to a spacious, airy duplex
in a brownstone with an actual backyard. That the yard was
covered in cement and the size of a prison cell mattered very
little; we bought a fifties-style glider from a junk store and an-
ticipated rocking there in the afternoons with Jess and staring
at the scraggly rosebushes that climbed a cracked wall at the
end of the "garden."

Our neighbor to the left was Nellie, a spry octogenarian
who always screeched a warning to me when I needed to

move my car before the cops ticketed it. To the right of us were Bill and his wife, a middle-aged couple of characters. Bill raised homing pigeons as a hobby. Smiling gappily, bereft of upper teeth, he introduced his wife as Harriet. She ignored him, took a deep drag on her thin, ladylike cigarette and, exhaling like a dragoness, said in a basso voice, "That's not my name." I was so taken aback at the time that I never could remember her real name. Bill was a great neighbor. Despite his earth-shattering sneezes that woke Jesse from a sound sleep even from next door, he was a thoughtful, generous man who took pains to let Jesse hold his precious pigeons and brought me unwanted dinners when Chris was away. Chris's career had picked up; we could now afford a decent apartment but he was away on location for months at a time.

Jesse was turning five, and ready for kindergarten at the nearby public school, Calabro Elementary, in the fall. My dogged research had yielded results; I discovered the New Jersey Statewide Parent Advocacy Network (SPAN), an organization that was parent-run and devoted to special-needs kids. It provided desperately needed information on kids with disabilities and inclusion in the public schools—the federal mandate for a "free and appropriate public education," in a regular classroom, with an aide and a curriculum adapted for the child's disability. This mandate was a result of the 1975 Individuals with Disabilities Education Act; it was still unfunded more than ten years later and still only spottily put into practice, with some states more successful than others and some districts ignoring it completely, despite the law being on the books.

I also learned about the Individualized Education Program

(IEP). It is supposed to be a blueprint jointly designed by parents and school administrators, laying out in detail the child's educational goals and how they would be attained. Parents are usually fighting for services to be delivered for their child: speech, occupational and sometimes physical therapies, one-on-one aides, adapted curriculum, and other ways to make school a success. This detailed outline must be signed by both the parents and the school administrators, and if nothing is agreed upon, the initial dispute can progress to mediation and, if that falls apart, a lawsuit. The IEP is a battle plan, but sometimes it causes war. Kindergarten was still a few months off, and that spring we enjoyed our new apartment and tried not to think of the possible wars to come.

We were on the swings every day in the little park a few blocks from our apartment. Jesse sat in my lap, shrieking and kicking as I pumped higher and higher. The park was a green oasis in urban Hoboken, with a sweet little bandstand in its center and a kiddie pool that had blue cement dolphins spraying water on hyperactive toddlers in the warm months. A short, pretty woman in her thirties stood nearby talking to her friend in Spanish. When the friend left, she lingered, smiling at Jess. We began a conversation; she told me, in heavily accented English, that her ten-year-old son was mentally challenged and went to the Calabro School, in a segregated classroom. She lived in the projects, far from the orderly brownstones that lined the main streets of Hoboken. We discussed the Hoboken child study team and her son's IEP. She was very unhappy with his placement in the school; she feared for his safety and complained that he wasn't learning anything, even life skills. I was taken aback when she told me in her uncertain English, "They give me the IEP to sign." I wasn't sure I understood.

"A completed IEP?"

She nodded.

"But you work with them to develop the program, right?"

She looked at me blankly.

"It's your right to be an equal partner with the team. You work together to develop the IEP," I told her.

I took her address and gave her mine, along with my phone number. Then I called the parent group and asked for a copy of a model IEP and a handbook for parents, along with a pamphlet in Spanish that spelled out her rights. When the material arrived, I brought it to her apartment, a grim cement cell in a warren of buildings, with missing light fixtures and litter in the hallways. We arranged for her to come to my place so I could write a letter for her to the Special Education Director outlining her son's needs and her request to reconvene the child study team so they could develop a new IEP.

I had my own meeting scheduled with the Hoboken child study team. Even if your child is bused to another district thirty miles away, as the team had suggested for Jesse's preschool, the child study team is always attached to the school system in the town or city where you live. The "team" usually includes a psychologist, a social worker, a special-needs teacher, and sometimes a school administrator, such as the principal.

The only team I had ever been on was Our Lady's junior varsity basketball team, and that had ended badly. I tended to get bored in the middle of games and space out, and someone had hurled a basketball at me during one game. My arms didn't even lift for it as I turned, still dazed, and the basketball hit my face, slamming my mouth, smashing my lips into my braces. My only memories of being on a team involved blood and pain, not to mention humiliation.

Those memories weren't far off from what my experience with various child study teams throughout Jesse's education would be, minus the actual blood. I hated being on a team, especially one that had to do with my son. I hated the sound of the word *team*, and its sports connotation. The word implied that we were merry mates all pulling together for Jesse, when in actuality, I felt like I was the one doing all the heavy lifting.

The team meetings usually began with a recitation of Jesse's limitations, a dour litany that felt like the assignment of blame. Then someone, usually the social worker, would lay out the school's plan for Jesse. During one meeting, I asked about including Jesse in a regular kindergarten class instead of segregating him. There was a pause. The social worker tried to be firm.

"There are the other parents. They might complain."

I was incredulous. "They might *complain?*"

There it was again, that basketball slamming my face.

She didn't look at me. She spoke directly to the files on the table before her. "Yes, well, Jesse will need extra attention."

"That's what Bernadette is for. She'll be there every day."

The social worker began a long description of the segregated program, but she didn't use the word *segregated*. She talked about how it would be much more beneficial for Jesse's special needs, but it still sounded like segregation to me. I launched accusingly into a description of my meeting with the

Mexican mother from the park, how disappointed she was with her son's placement, and how she didn't even know she could have input into the IEP.

The social worker tried to reassure me, saying, "Oh, Mrs. Cooper, you're not like that other element."

Her words took my breath away. But it was just a momentary ebb. I felt a riptide of rage begin to flow through me.

"What? The nonwhite element? But I have more in common with them than with you. Your name ends in a vowel, and you"—I pointed at the psychologist—"are Irish-American. Fifty years ago, *you* were 'that other element.'"

The social worker got very busy putting her papers in order and changed the subject. The psychologist stared at me like he had found a new subject for a research article on displaced anger and mothers of disabled children in extreme denial.

The meeting ended with a tentative IEP and provision for speech and occupational therapy services for Jesse in a segregated classroom. I was to take this proposal home, study it with Chris, and return it signed and approved for Jesse's fall class at the Calabro School kindergarten. No other option was offered. I was unhappy about that, but resigned because I was unclear about how to get Jesse into a regular classroom. He was still small, and this was only kindergarten, I told myself. First grade would be the time to reconsider inclusion in a regular classroom with his able-bodied peers.

September approached, and I received a notice in the mail for another meeting that I assumed was to hammer out the final details of Jesse's program. It was an early-morning meeting with a strange time slot: 8:00 to 8:15 a.m. When I arrived at the school, I found a roomful of special-needs parents, all frantically checking their watches, terrified of being late for work, all waiting for their kids' IEPs to be rubber-stamped by the child study team. Everyone had the same time slot for the same meeting. They were being taken in the order in which they arrived, like people at a supermarket checkout line. I scanned the worried faces of the parents in the room. No one deserved this assembly-line treatment.

I walked into the special education director's office without knocking.

"What you are doing right now is reprehensible," I said, in a voice louder than I intended.

I stood there, a quaking aspen trying to pass as a redwood.

"Sit down, Mrs. Cooper."

So I can be shorter than you, I thought.

"No thank you. I'm only here to say this: either you get the New Jersey parent group for special needs in to talk to these parents and explain their rights or I'm going to the newspaper and telling them how taxpayers are treated in Hoboken. I'll call your office with the number of the parent group."

I walked out the door, still shaking inside.

A new, radicalized self was emerging, midwifed by injustice.

Jesse was placed in the segregated kindergarten at Calabro School that fall, with Bernadette as his aide. Jesse was the only physically disabled kid in his class; all the others had learning disabilities or hyperactive syndromes. His teacher was a dedicated, kind woman who regularly brought in fresh fruit to supplement the overly sugared breakfasts provided by the state for her students. Despite my letters to the press and repeated phone calls to the special ed director, I hadn't been able to effect any noticeable change in the business-as-usual world of special education in Hoboken. The mothers I had met, like the Mexican mother in the park, were afraid of retribution if they complained.

Jesse's IEP mandated a speech therapist, Eleanor, who was positive and upbeat; Jesse loved her and performed well in her sessions. Bernadette took notes; every day I eagerly read about Jesse's progress: "Repeated 'go out' several times; said words 'down,' 'okay,' 'hand.'"

I visited Jesse's class regularly and was happy to see that the children were learning songs, colors, the alphabet, seasons, and more, but I was beginning to dread first grade. Would Jesse be separated from his nondisabled peers for his entire elementary school experience? The regular classrooms for the upper grades were overcrowded; I often heard frustrated teachers yelling when I walked in the halls. I wasn't hopeful that things would improve by the next year. I began to search for a place to live that might actually implement inclusion, even if it meant uprooting us and moving to another state.

In the meantime, our financial upswing meant that we could expand therapies for Jesse. We found an alternative therapist, Cheryl, who was a Feldenkrais practitioner in nearby Nutley, New Jersey. Feldenkrais is a gentle, noninvasive therapy that "teaches" the nervous system to redirect growth and gain awareness through movement, using the nervous system's ability to change and learn. Cheryl, a tiny woman in her thirties with a mop of curly hair, manipulated Jesse's limbs while engaging his mind, encouraging his awareness of where his body was in space. "You're sitting! Do you feel that? You're sitting on your butt, little man!"

Jesse responded very well to Cheryl's manipulations; she was invariably upbeat and cheered on Jesse's small triumphs, although I have a hilarious photograph of one of her sessions that looks otherwise. Jesse is sitting on the therapy table and Cheryl is holding onto both his hands for balance. She looks directly at him with a huge encouraging smile but Jesse's face is turned to the camera with a pout so exaggerated he looks like a Greek tragedy mask. Generally, though, Jesse's moments of tragedy were few with Cheryl; Bernadette and I drove Jesse to Nutley twice a week, and we paid out of pocket for Cheryl's services.

Feldenkrais therapy was paying off. At our next yearly visit to our pediatrician, Dr. Joe Rocchio, he commented on how limber Jesse felt to him. Dr. Joe had been Jesse's pediatrician since his days in the NICU. He was living proof that not all members of the medical profession were androids, and the only doctor we looked forward to visiting. At our first appointment, he stunned me by picking Jess up, kissing him, and proclaiming, "*Look* at this beautiful boy! Look at him!"

Dr. Joe put up with my quirks, wisecracking when I climbed onto the table and nursed Jesse while he gave him his immunizations; I in turn put up with his little secret: he smoked, and I often let him light up at the end of an appointment. He sat across his desk, savoring his smoke, a skinny little man only as tall as I, with an oversized nose, acne scars from his adolescent years, and a shock of thick black hair: not at all conventionally good-looking, his dark eyes piercing and his manner sarcastic, all to mask a too tender heart.

I adored him for being so loving to Jesse, and for being instantly available when I called him, frantic over fevers and colds. I called him once from Santa Fe so panicked I could barely blurt out what happened. Jesse had rolled off the hotel bed and onto the floor, which was lushly carpeted—he was totally unharmed, but I needed to hear Dr. Joe tell me that. I am grateful to him for those human sparks that lit my way in a wilderness of loss and confusion. And I am indebted to him for introducing me to a woman who would change my life.

At that yearly exam in Joe's Greenwich Village office, Joe handled Jesse lovingly, as always, but this time he wanted to know what was going on.

"What are you doing with him, Mrs. Goldberg?" (He amused himself by calling me ever-varying nicknames.) "He looks great!"

I told him about the Feldenkrais therapy.

"Listen, do me a favor. I'm going to give you a number to call—Mary Somoza. She's the mother of twin girls with cerebral palsy. Will you tell her about this therapy?"

I would do anything for Joe, so I called. My first conversation with Mary was only about Feldenkrais therapy and the Sisyphean efforts of getting therapy services for our kids, but she soon became a lifelong mentor and friend. Mary was a veteran of respite care wars and her competence and organization were almost intimidating at first. Her honesty and humanity still move me today.

Mary Mooney Somoza was born in Dublin, raised in England, and living in Spain when she met her future husband,

Gerardo Somoza, on a visit to New York City. She lived on Fifty-seventh Street in Manhattan with Gerardo and four children in a two-story walk-up. Every day she hefted two wheelchairs up and down those narrow stairs. Alba and Anastasia, her twins, both had severe cerebral palsy. Anastasia was verbal, Alba nonverbal. Mary and Gerardo also had a boy, Oliver, two years older than the twins, and a girl, Gabriella, two years younger. The twins were about eight years old when I first met Mary.

Mary became an advocate out of sheer necessity. Money was tight and she had four kids, two of them disabled. Her husband was a freelance photographer. Dr. Joe had tended all of her children since birth, including making home visits, and had never charged her a dime. Mary was a fighter. She was already known in New York City as a relentless voice for respite care at home to avoid institutionalization, and she had changed laws for the disabled. She advocated for her girls with a combination of ferocious tenacity and irresistible Irish charm.

After our first phone conversation, I watched a documentary about her family shown in Hoboken. On-screen, Mary was a vibrant, beautiful woman with a range of emotions that mirrored my own. I saw her hefting her daughter's wheelchair up a narrow stairway, charming legislators in Albany, and, in a scene that left me in tears, washing and cuddling Alba in the early morning before a surgery for her hip dislocation due to spasticity. In a heart-searing moment Mary looks into the camera and speaks honestly about her fears for the surgery. She says she thought about what would happen if she lost Alba, and that she actually thought "there would be less work" for an instant of time before she realized what she was thinking. "I said, God, give me all the work in the world, but let me have Alba. She's . . . my special one."

I called her immediately after seeing the documentary, now knowing she was a soul mate. In that conversation, I told her about my fears for Jesse's educational future in Hoboken. She still remembers what I said to her.

"I can stay here and be Joan of Arc of Hoboken or we can move to Massachusetts, where inclusion of disabled kids is better than the national average."

Chris and I began to make pro and con lists. Could we survive as artists outside New York or Los Angeles? We had lived in an urban setting for seventeen years. Could we live in a small town after seventeen years of in-your-face city life? Could we even afford to buy a house? We considered upstate New York, Nyack, and the little town in Massachusetts where I had spent summers by the ocean with Aunt Ellie and Uncle Benny. We studied our pro and con lists. One line about Massachusetts that made both columns was "family close by."

We were leaning toward New England. There were world-famous hospitals there, old friends, and the promise of better schools. In Massachusetts, I would be effectively giving up acting and concentrating on writing. But I thought I could do it, and get as much joy from creating a script as an individual character. Chris was working on locations all over the United States. And that meant we could live anywhere. In this way, Jesse freed us. All those years of looking at cement transoms as my limited vista were about to become what I only saw in yearning dreams. I would now be looking at and smelling salt water again. I was going home.

When I picture leaving Hoboken, I see Bill smiling his jack-o'-lantern smile and waving good-bye, Harriet beside him in a head-obscuring cloud of cigarette smoke. I hear the pigeons murmuring in worried undertones that echo my own misgivings. We pull out of our prized parking space near the brownstone, the one Nellie's sharp eyes scored for us, and drive our packed Toyota past the little parks, the Italian grocery stores, the Malibu Diner, and the Calabro Elementary School. We enter the Lincoln Tunnel and come out on the other side of our lives.

Jesse was entering first grade in September. We moved to Massachusetts in July.

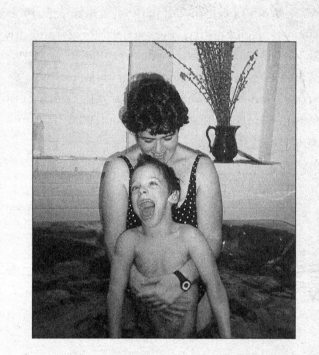

Suzanne and Jesse, age six, in the hot tub

CHAPTER THIRTEEN

St. Suzanne of Cork and Dymphna the Doleful

One of the hardest things about leaving Hoboken and moving to our small town in Massachusetts was leaving Bernadette. She wanted to stay near New York and realize her life's dream of nursing. Thankfully, she handpicked a young woman named Suzanne to be her successor. We knew Suzanne would be with us only for the first phase of our life in this new town; she was engaged to a Scotsman and would move to Glasgow at the end of our year together. Suzanne would be the first of Jesse's tender women to be living with us, and she came along for the move from Hoboken in July of 1994. Her fiancé, Donald, and his brother from Scotland were visiting and helped us move into our boxy raised ranch, which seemed to us like Xanadu after years of living in cramped apartments.

The downstairs of our new house gave Suzanne a private space; she had her own room and bath, but she easily made the transition into the mainstream of our home. She loved my jet fuel coffee, having nannied with a French family before us, and had an appreciation for our Mediterranean cooking. Best of all, her wry humor fitted perfectly with ours, especially Jesse's.

That first summer, Suzanne would take a "wee walk" with Jesse every day down to the marina, which was at the end of our street. On the way, they would pass a small cedar-shingled house belonging to a lonely old man who cultivated roses and had developed a huge crush on Suzanne. She gave a running commentary as they approached the house every day.

"Oh, Jaysus, Jesse, he's spotted us."

The old man came running out of the house, holding a rose.

"I think he lurks behind the curtains waiting for us, Jess. Let's speed up."

Jesse would caw, knowingly. The old man bestowed the rose on Suzanne.

"Oh, brilliant, thanks so much. I'll tell my *fiancé* I got a beautiful rose today."

And off they'd sprint to the marina, succumbing to giggles once they were out of sight.

Suzanne was tall, with soft, vulnerable features and short, thick, coal-black hair. Her low-pitched voice had the musical accent of Rebel Cork, which had birthed some of the fiercest fighters in Ireland's long struggle against its British oppressors. As calm and maternal as she appeared, Suzanne had that rebel spirit, too, an inner strength and resilience that gave her the fortitude to abide with our daily struggles. She was in her early twenties, athletic and strong, and thought nothing of cycling five miles to the mall. When I protested that I would drive her anywhere she liked on her days off, she just laughed.

"Tch. Marianne, I'm Irish."

She never explained what that meant. To me, it meant that she had overcome far greater problems in her life than a five-mile bike ride to get where she wanted to go. Despite her ready and easy laugh, Suzanne harbored a melancholy that came of an unhappy childhood, one that involved periodic financial instability from a father who liked to gamble and the sorrows that came with that scenario. Out of this tinge of sadness grew a compassion that reached out to Jesse, a sheltering impulse that selflessly gave comfort where she had had none.

Jesse relaxed into Suzanne, bobbing blissfully against her full bosom in the hot tub we had installed for him in the corner of the big room downstairs, shrieking happily when she pushed him on his special swing we brought from Hoboken. And Suzanne nestled into our family, too, plopping down on our oversized red couch to watch movies with us at night after Jesse went to sleep, savoring the Italian foods my mother made at family gatherings. She missed her fiancé, though, and sometimes spent half her weekly wages on transatlantic phone calls with him, planning their future together in Scotland.

After Suzanne left us the following spring to begin her new life in Glasgow, I lost touch with her. Then, in a flash of the synchronicity that has colored my life these last few years, she called me just as I was beginning to tell her story in these pages. She had gone online to find out what films Chris had recently made and had discovered the news of Jesse's death. She was calling to express her shock, her sympathy.

She lives in Ireland now because the younger of her two sons has been diagnosed with Asperger's syndrome, a form of autism, and she says the Irish are more accepting of children who are "different." I'm not surprised. Both Suzanne and Bernadette always saw Jesse the kid, not the disability. I thought it must come from somewhere in their culture, the same one that nurtured brilliant quadriplegic writers like Christy Brown and Christopher Nolan. Suzanne's year with Jesse was a prologue to her own story, and her tenderness has been overlaid with steely resolve as she fights for her own boy and his place in the world, Jesse's spirit guiding her, I hope.

After Suzanne left, our family was again in a quandary. Chris was due to leave for Texas to shoot another John Sayles film, and I would be a single mother again all summer. The New York–based *Irish Echo* was no help in Massachusetts. Finally, I found a service headed by a nun, Sister Veronica—which should have been my first warning—that led me to Jesse's next caregiver, Dymphna. (Dymphna is not her real name; I have named her for the Irish saint who is patron of the mentally ill.)

When I picture Dymphna now, I see a kewpie doll–faced woman in her twenties, careless of her appearance, slumped in a lawn chair smoking a cigarette and desultorily pushing Jesse in his swing. She was always depressed. I found out why after not too long: a priest in her hometown had sexually abused her. When she reported it to her family, their response was to institutionalize her in a place where they prescribed electro-shock treatments.

I can picture it: "The priest took advantage of you? *You must be crazy.*"

Years later, when I saw *The Magdalene Sisters,* an Irish film about unwed mothers brutalized by lifelong incarceration in a laundry run by the church for profit, I was not surprised by the wholesale cruelty Dymphna suffered. A character in the film was being serially raped by a priest; she was taken from the home in the middle of the night and placed in an institution.

I had seen the results of this kind of inhumanity in my own home while Dymphna lived with us. There was no breezy Suzanne-style plopping down on furniture while Dymphna was living with us. Anger gnawed just at the edge of her conscious-ness, but she was passive, listless around us all. I picked up on her buried anger and began to feel tentative in my own home. Jesse was subdued. The arrangement wasn't working. Jesse's mojo that called angels to us had now drawn a damaged one.

Dymphna was someone who did not see Jesse as a child of God because she didn't see herself as one. The bruising of her soul had left a mark, and she was unable to see beyond her own pain. I felt guilty, but I wanted her gone. For Jesse, for me. We couldn't help heal her, and she couldn't help Jesse. After only two months, I gave Dymphna her notice. The only good thing that came out of Dymphna's hasty departure was that it opened the door for Jesse's next caregiver, Brandy, who stayed with us ten years, until Jess left us.

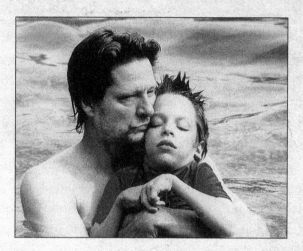

Chris and Jesse, age six, in the pool

When I swim I feel

Remarkable

Mellow

To me, swimming is when I feel;

When I swim I feel

To me swimming is

Powerful

Liberating

When I swim I feel

—*Jesse Cooper*

CHAPTER FOURTEEN

Pod People

I am coated in dust and memories. Every day Chris and I go out to the two giant metal storage pods in our driveway and sort through their musty contents. They have been sitting here for nine months, during the total renovation of the lower level of our home, and are stuffed chockablock with fourteen years of accumulated stuff.

Fourteen years of living in this house on a tidal river, in this characterless raised ranch that Jesse turned into a giant magnet, drawing friends and family into a swirling maelstrom of love and food and shrieks of laughter and screams of triumph and despair, all because he was there at the heart's core of the house. Fourteen years of things, every one resonating with a certain time, a certain place. We're not moving, but we're moving on. Everything will change. But I hate change, and I hate Chris for instigating this one.

For a second I think I could just live in the pods, like Miss Havisham at her ruined wedding feast. I could clear a space to my old wicker rocker crammed at the back of the pod, the one I've had since college and used to sit in with Jess. I could sit there and defy the passage of time, ignoring the cobwebs hanging from Jess's Buzz Lightyear bank and the dusty boxes of schoolwork and medical files and unproduced screenplays and family pictures and Chris's acting awards and my kitschy religious artifacts.

No. I have to get to work.

I open a box and a big, messy envelope with "Ma's roses" scrawled across the top is the first thing I see. Oh, yeah. I was supposed to have the flowers at her wake made into rosary beads. Sorry, Ma.

I find a play I wrote when I was seventeen, called *Escape to Gynt*. Everyone in it is a pseudo-intellectual and they all drown in sewage at the end. All except our heroine, "Joan," whom we first meet strumming a dulcimer on the bathroom floor and wearing a monk's cowl. She is not a pseudo—which I pronounced "sway-dough" at the time—intellectual. She has "scars on her wrists." After I stop laughing, I realize I am hardwired for morbidity. ("Scars on her wrists"? Rosary beads from funeral flowers?)

At the bottom of a pile of schoolwork, I find Jesse's last essay for his sophomore English class, dated November 30, 2004.

COURAGE

by Jesse Cooper

Courage is an attribute that allows you to face difficulty and danger with firmness and without fear. Atticus Finch said on page 112 of *To Kill a Mockingbird* that courage is "knowing you're licked before you begin but you begin anyway and you see it through no matter what. . . . "

I knew I was licked before this renovation began, but I have to see it through no matter what.

▦

The bottom half of our house is laid out exactly the same as the top half: two small rooms, a small bathroom, and a big open room, as well as a small second kitchen and laundry room. When Jesse was alive the downstairs bedroom directly below ours belonged to Suzanne, then Dymphna, then Brandy. There was a small bathroom under our upstairs bathroom, and I had a small office under Jesse's upstairs bedroom. The open room was Jesse's weekend hangout, with a big-screen TV, a leather couch, and a puffy beanbag chair. The room opened onto the indoor pool, an enclosed room we built under the upstairs deck.

In November, the downstairs was gutted to the studs and became unrecognizable. Workmen and dust swarmed into the house, and every day an earsplitting Dropkick Murphys soundtrack screamed along with the hammering and electric drills. Even Jesse's indoor pool has been removed. We have no more need for one that sticks halfway out of the ground; we won't be lifting Jesse into it anymore. The new exercise pool will be sunk into the ground, six feet deep, with a nifty cover that rolls back with the flip of a switch. The only one using it will most likely be me, treading water, an irony that makes me smirk at how life can hurl corny metaphors at you: I'm barely keeping my head above water these days.

I'd rather dive below the surface of my thoughts and remember the old pool, one gloomy Sunday in November when Chris is away and Jesse and I are alone. I lug the heavy gray covers off one by one—there are three of them, in sections. I test the water. Jesse is fifteen, waiting patiently in his wheelchair. I lift him out of it, grunting with effort, and lay him down on the table beside the pool. He doesn't weigh much, maybe seventy pounds, but he is all gangly arms and legs that stick out stiffly, sometimes catching on my own arms or legs. I retrieve Jesse's neck float, move him to a sitting position, and awkwardly fit on the float with one hand, supporting his back with the other. I smile at him. He smiles back, anticipating the delight to come. I lift him under his arms and heave him over the side of the pool.

He yelps happily at the sensation of water and weightlessness as the chains of gravity drop away. His tight muscles relax and he kicks his legs. I hold up a CD for his approval. "Nelly Furtado?" He clicks "yes." I climb in. We float. Nelly sings, "I'm like a bird, I'll only fly away." I get really close to Jesse, eye to eye, and we stare at each other until one of us laughs. I am not afraid of the time when I will have to lift him out of the pool, in an hour or so. I am strong and I know I can do it. I can do anything for Jess. I have courage.

▣

Now, back inside the house, I realize that Chris too has courage, because he designed and pushed forward this renovation. He knew it was time to use the entire house. He loves renovating homes; it was his day job before he became a full-time actor. When we first moved here, he put in a new roof, wainscoted the walls of our bedroom, restored an antique cedar chest and a huge oak table. He designed and planned every detail of the renovation with painstaking measurements and lines on graph paper.

Still, only a few weeks into the renovation, Chris wept as he told me of a dream he had had. Jesse's caregiver Brandy was in her former bedroom and she had put everything back: chairs, bed, nightstands. She uncovered a blanket on her lap and Jesse sat up, laughing. A joke on Dad: I'm still here! His telling me the dream makes me forgive Chris for pushing us to change.

I know Jess is still here in our home, but I need courage, too, as the renovation is completed. Jesse's room doesn't look like his anymore, now that all the rooms have been changed around. We sleep downstairs now and Jess's bed is in our old room, which has been transformed into a guest room. Jesse's room looks different with Brandy's bed in it. Standing in it now, I see that the antique dark wood double bed makes the hang-

ing dolphin mobile and Jesse's posters look weird. They are
too kidlike for this newly grown-up room, silly blue dolphins
dancing in the wind against the somber dark wood of the antique bed.

I reach up to unhook the mobile from the ceiling. My arm
falls to my side. I try to take down the dolphin mobile three
times and fail. Finally I leave it there, along with the League of
Pissed-Off Voters and Lord of the Rings posters. I've lost count
of how many times I've cried today.

I move to leave the room but notice Jesse's blue slipper
socks hiding in plain sight, tucked into his bookcase. As I
stroke them for comfort, they remind me of Albert, the handsome twenty-two-year-old from Cameroon who helped us on
Saturdays. We were thrilled to have Albert because aside from
Chris, Jesse was often surrounded by women. Now Jesse and
his best friend Kyle had another guy near their age to hang out
with on weekends.

Albert brought them both to a place they had never been,
showing them on a globe where he was born, and telling them
stories of growing up in Cameroon, a moon away from our
icy New England town. But he laughed as hard as they did
at Jim Carrey movies and ate just as much pizza, sprawled on
the couch, bending over occasionally to straighten Jesse on his
beanbag chair.

Shy and cautious with Chris and me, Albert was voluble
with Jess and Kyle. One day I overheard a deep discussion
on the afterlife, the squeaks of the glider on the deck punc-
tuating Jesse's clicks and Albert's soft deep voice. That same

velvety voice always pronounced Jesse's name with an elongated chuckle underneath, the soft, strange vowels sounding a familiar song. His strong, sure hands lifted Jesse easily into the pool or massaged his tight legs and feet with a tenderness that was almost prayerful. Jess received easily his quiet strength and gentle spirit; the closest men in his life represented those qualities: his dad, Uncle Benny, Uncle Mike, Uncle Gary.

Rubbing Jesse's slipper socks brings me back to the day following Jesse's death, the house thronged with people. I found Albert alone in Jesse's room holding a single sock. His silent tears dropped onto the soft wool that had recently warmed Jesse's feet, turning the light blue into the color of loss.

I take Jesse's pillow for my new bed downstairs, the pillow I carefully hid from Chris all these months because I didn't want him to wash it. It's the last place Jesse's head touched. It has his dried saliva on the pillowcase. This is how deranged I am now. I'm saving dried saliva from my son. I quickly rip off the pillowcase like a Band-Aid on a sore and put it in the wash. I put the freshly covered pillow on my new bed. Maybe Jesse will give me a dream, too, where he's laughing about my fear of taking down the dolphins and my madness in preserving his saliva and petting his socks.

Instead Jesse gives me treasure. I found a digital camera's memory chip in the pods, in the corner of a cardboard box, a tiny piece of ephemera, easily overlooked. I have no idea what's on it, but the next day I venture out to CVS and on the photo machine, I see Jesse at sixteen, shining like an avatar from another world. His beautiful face is suffused with light because the shot is overexposed—a sure sign I was the one wielding the camera. He has a world-weary expression, mandatory in the don't-bug-me-with-photos teenage lexicon.

He's flashing the new gold earring on his left ear, the one he got pierced for his second-to-last birthday. Brandy took him to the piercing place at the mall, along with Kyle and Jamie, and they returned triumphantly to surprise me with Jesse's new look. The day had been filled with drama, and they bounded through the house, limbs flying, squealing like puppies as they reported it.

The woman at the first place dismissed Jesse after looking down at him in his wheelchair, and flatly refused to pierce his ear. Kyle and Jamie were outraged. The group retreated to the food court, fuming. Brandy treated everyone to junk food, savored all the more by Jesse because it was usually forbidden.

Fortified by burritos, they sallied forth to another store, a determined team. The young woman at this place was happy to pierce Jesse's ear. Jamie giggled as she told me they had gone back to the first place and walked back and forth, loudly praising Jesse's new earring. Kyle chimed in, laughing about how ridiculous they all were. The first woman hadn't even noticed them, but they still felt triumphant, like they had fought a battle together and won.

"And Jesse was so brave! When that other girl pierced his ear he didn't even flinch!" Kyle squeaked.

I looked at Jesse, warrior boy. He gave me that cool, nonchalant look that is in the picture I hold in my hands. And I am so happy that for a moment I forget to hate the present change.

Now the pods are empty and I'm over my resentment of

the renovation and its spillover to Chris. I lie on Jesse's pillow in our new room, in our new bed, and I look at the tidal river outside my window from another perspective. The room is beautiful, elegant. The river seems closer somehow. And I got the dream, a bonus gift from Jess. In it, I couldn't find Jesse. One minute I was feeding him beside the oak table, the next minute he was gone. Then I reached under the daybed and touched his warm flesh. He slid out from under the daybed, smiling a smile that stays with me for the whole day.

Courage is like one ant trying to cross a roaring stream. It may seem impossible but you have to try.

—*Jesse Cooper*

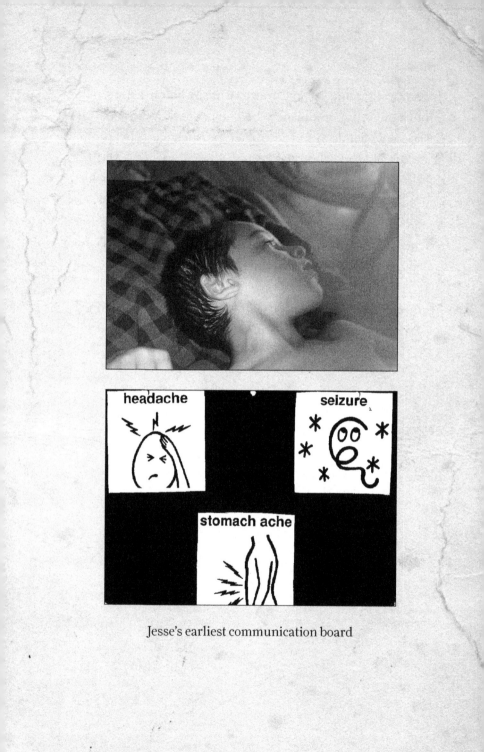

Jesse's earliest communication board

CHAPTER FIFTEEN

Puppet

Journal, 1990: *It's definitely the seizures that have made me so convinced he'll die. They look so brutal, so demonic, the way they suddenly possess him in the middle of a laugh, a kick or a spoonful of food, turning him into a helpless puppet with a frozen look of fear in his eyes staring from a distorted face, one that was beautiful only a second ago.*

Special diets. Magnets. Phenobarbital. Klonopin. Dilantin. Valium. Tegretol. Neurontin. Biofeedback. Acupuncture. Craniosacral therapy. Herbs. Vitamins. Amino acids. Reiki. Holy water from Ireland. Crystals. The anti-*malocchio*. Prayer. Spells. Cursing the fates.

Nothing worked.

Jesse had generalized tonic-clonic seizures that lasted from one to two minutes. What Jesse didn't have: status epilepticus, where a person stops breathing and goes into a seizure that doesn't end; the kind of seizures that destroy short-term memory and affect cognition; the kind of seizures that are brought on by flashing lights. Jesse never knew a day in his life without seizures—even in the neonatal intensive care unit, his brain scans showed seizure activity. He came home from the hospital with antiseizure drugs coloring his formula a sickly pink.

A dark seizure god ruled Jesse. And us. We never knew when a sunny bout of giggles would be interrupted and Jesse would be jerked away, his invisible strings pulled by the puppetmaster of his broken brain circuitry. Sometimes it would be only a two-second startle, just enough of a poke to remind us that Jesse's life wasn't his own. Sometimes it would last as long as two minutes, full-blown, his body stiffening, his limbs flailing, little *uh-uh-uh* distress shrieks coming from his tightened lips, his eyes crazed and rolling. Instinct made me cover his body with mine, clasping him to me, trying to stop it through sheer will, chanting "okayokayokayokay," while inside my head incoherent screams competed to drown out his cries. Sometimes it was as if he experienced a thrill, and he would giggle afterward, but the giggles were tainted, seizure giggles, sinister, someone else's giggles, not Jesse's. Sometimes he would fall afterward into a deep, deathlike sleep.

When Jesse was an infant I loved nursing him beyond all reason. It was the one thing I controlled in a world where Jesse otherwise belonged to medical professionals. It was something I could do for him to help him survive. It was shared bliss to hold him so close, to inhale his singular scent, to see him look up and smile, sated. I pumped breast milk for the seven weeks he was in the neonatal intensive care unit, but I also gave him formula, against the dark mutterings of the La Leche League, who said he would then refuse the breast. They were wrong about that, as was the neonatologist who warned me he would be too weak to nurse. Jesse latched on while still in the NICU, and continued to nurse with gusto until the day I was forced to give it up. A neurologist had suggested the ketogenic diet, a high-fat, adequate-protein, low-carb diet that effectively starves the body to produce ketosis, an anticonvulsant effect.

The diet twisted Jesse's little guts and made him writhe in pain, a gastrointestinal nightmare that made colic look like a walk in the park.

We visited neurologist after neurologist. Each had his or her drug of choice, and every drug came with side effects almost more frightening to us than the seizures. Our worries increased when we learned that the FDA does not test drugs on children under twelve. We knew that people reacted differently to different drugs, but Jesse seemed to be acutely sensitive to any kind of medication. When he was medicated to undergo a CT scan, he slept long past the time he should have awakened and even the neonatologist looked worried.

Another neurologist, Dr. D., prescribed phenobarbital for his seizures, which made him sleep all day. In 1990 the *New York Times* published an article about phenobarbital, saying it was "ineffective and perhaps harmful." To our surprise, they quoted Dr. D. saying that physicians are often the ones who respond to parental pressure to prescribe phenobarbital because they were afraid of seizures. Chris and I had seen Jesse's seizures, and they weren't as frightening as the stuff I was reading in the *Physician's Desk Reference* about the drugs Jesse had been prescribed.

Dr. D. wanted to give Jesse ACTH, a steroid. I thought it was too dangerous—a partial list of some "common" side effects were abnormal hair growth on body or face, easily angered or annoyed, Cushing's syndrome—symptoms of which include muscle weakness, psychosis, hypertension, etc., etc.—all the way through a Hieronymus Bosch portrait of things that could go wrong with a human body. Dr. D. said that I felt that way because I was "from the sixties, and overreacting to drug use." Really? Vanity alone would have precluded my use of pot at the age of nineteen if the common side effects were abnormal hair growth all over my face and body, or even one-tenth of the laundry list of medical horrors attached as side effects to the medication Dr. D. wanted to prescribe.

The next neurologist prescribed Dilantin (phenytoin sodium). Dilantin's side effects included coarsening of facial features and hirsutism, both of which Jesse never developed, thankfully. Instead he had agonizing months of teething while on Dilantin, which hardened his gums and made every new tooth a dagger of pain. Klonopin (clonazepam) worked for only a month, which is why it's called the "honeymoon" drug. Tegretol (carbamazepine) put him in the hospital with an adverse reaction contrary to the long list of possible side effects. Instead of being lethargic on Tegretol, Jesse was bouncing off the walls—and in such medical danger that his then neurologist ordered him hospitalized after a random, unscheduled blood test for something else. Then Jesse was put on yet another drug, I forget which one. It didn't matter. None of them worked. When the doctors were honest, they admitted that they really didn't know how the brain functioned. Nor, specifically, did they know how Jesse's brain worked or why he had seizures. They thought the seizures were caused by misdirected electrical signals bouncing off scar tissue in his brain from the bleed he had when he was four days old, but other children suffered the same severity of cerebral hemorrhage without seizures. The doctors also didn't know how Jesse would react to all the different drugs they prescribed. It was all a wait-and-see crapshoot, with an emergency trip to the hospital if it all went wrong. We only trusted the doctors who admitted they didn't really know.

Eventually, we took Jesse off all drugs, and, with the approval of Jesse's last neurologist, Dr. Thiele, we used one half of a five-milligram Valium (diazepam) on days when he seemed distracted and twitchy and about to have a big seizure, and a larger dose when he did have a big one. It was dangerous to have him off drugs, and his past history showed it to be dangerous to have him on drugs. His seizures were never controlled.

I kept logs to see if the seizures were affected by diet, weather, emotion, flashing lights, sound, allergies, seasons. We saw a slight increase in seizure activity before a thunderstorm. We saw no increase when he went on rides at Universal Studios that warned of flashing lights. We saw no other discernible connection. When he was four, we taped magnets to a headband that he wore every day and he actually went without a twitch for two months. Then, inexplicably, the seizures started up again.

Nothing, nothing worked.

Jesse hated the seizures. He hated living on the fault line that would send him tumbling through space at the exact moment when, through sheer warrior fortitude, he would master some Herculean feat like writing a poem, or windsurfing, or playing a computer game. I asked him about it one day when he was about thirteen. His huge dark eyes held mine, his face serious and intent.

"Are the seizures the worst part of your disability?"

His eyes never leaving mine, he gave his most emphatic "click" for "yes."

"I hate them, too."

I did. I hated them, hated them, hated them, and I was right to hate them because they killed my child. But Jesse's neurologist told me that it was likely he didn't die from a seizure. He died when his brain told his heart to stop, she said. The exact cause was probably SUDEP, Sudden Unexplained Death in Epilepsy, which is not well understood, even by epilepsy professionals. But they do know that SUDEP is more likely to happen to people with uncontrolled seizure disorders.

No one had explained the possibility of SUDEP to us, his parents. We didn't know such a condition existed. But would we have been better off knowing that someday SUDEP could take Jesse? No, knowing the details wouldn't have mattered, because I knew. I always knew.

Someday I'll find him dead in his bed.

We were helpless to protect Jesse when he finally started spending more time away from us at school. I worried constantly that a panicked school nurse would summon the paramedics, who would arrive after the seizure was over, terrifying him with their sirens and bustle, rushing him to the hospital, where there was nothing to be done, except give him drugs after the fact. Fear of the seizures and their awful power colored every public moment, so that our pride and delight in seeing Jesse with his sixth-grade class at graduation had the ever-present undertone of fear that he would seize when he was onstage receiving his hard-earned diploma.

We never got used to the seizures, but we were well aware of how scary they looked to observers. They terrified us, too, but we knew they would be over in a minute. A horrifying minute where time became infinity. I became adept at wheeling Jesse out of rooms abruptly when he had seizures out in public view, or sheltering his body with mine if there was no immediate avenue of escape. We were trapped together, yet far apart, for those one or two minutes, frozen in a time-stop zone of misery and fear.

I began to leave my body when he left his. It was the only way to endure watching the seizures that possessed him like an ancient, malevolent force. When I turn on the news and see mothers watching their babies die during a famine, I know they are outside their bodies, too. It's all you can do when nothing works to stop your child from leaving you, and you can't keep him. How else can you look at their suffering? You have to leave. You become an outlier in a dead space, in a preview of the remote world where you will wander when he is not there permanently. And even though I was watching him seize from that faraway place, it wasn't enough of an escape. I wanted release from this horror—for Jesse and for me. I would think,

It would be better if he died. I even said to him, just once, on a horrible day of multiple prolonged seizures: "Jesse, you can go. I know you don't want this. I know you hate this. You can go." I feel no guilt about that, even now. Because even now, riven by loss, I exult that he will never, ever have another seizure.

After Jesse died from this fluke, this grotesquely named medical condition, after everyone went home and the house was a silent tomb, I opened the kitchen drawer and took out his seizure meds. I flung them into the trash. I cursed them. And then I actually felt something besides pain for the first time since Jesse died. I felt satisfaction. I slammed down the cover to the trash.

Fuck you. You never worked.

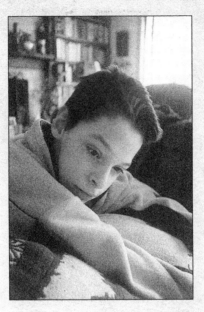

Jesse, age ten

"Cogito ergo sum" means "I think, therefore I am."
—Jesse's ninth grade Latin homework,
taken from his computer

CHAPTER SIXTEEN

Three Graces

My dealings with neurologists in the course of Jesse's medical life were always fraught with social dysfunction. On their side. I'm not the picture of mental health and admit that the towering grizzly mother part of my persona was always in the room with every member of the medical community who treated my son. But the mortal fear Chris and I felt about Jesse's seizures and their possible effect on his body and mental capacities was made worse by what felt like interspecies communication with doctors. Occasionally a neurologist would rise to the level of cyborg, if we were lucky, speaking in English instead of words we would have to look up later. Those were the ones who spoke only to Chris and me. But even when that happened, I stopped listening. While they droned on about "brain insults" and pushed wonder drugs that didn't work, I was having a shouted one-way conversation with them in my head.

"Can you see my son? He's sitting right here, in my lap.

"He is a sentient being, a member of the human race. Are you?

"His brain isn't just a meat computer that crashed with a fatal error.

"He is alive, conscious. Can you tell me where the seat of consciousness is? Is it in the brain?"

The conversation never went beyond the voices in my head. We just listened to their drug suggestions and brain insult descriptions and then moved on, insulted in our own way by the snubbing of Jesse's soul. Another office, another neurologist. We weren't shopping for a better prognosis. We knew Jesse had brain damage and a seizure disorder. We were looking for grace.

If we couldn't find a neurologist who could regenerate Jesse's damaged brain cells, could we at least find one who could show us some mercy and who had the moral strength to see Jesse as human?

We found three, all women.

I don't remember how I found the first, Dr. Catherine Spears, when Jesse was not yet two and in the throes of horrific teething pain. She was in her early seventies then and, unfortunately for us, about to retire. I remember thinking that at the time Dr. Spears went to medical school, she must have been the only woman specializing in the male-dominated field of neurology and that it took a strong temperament to withstand that particular trial by fire. Her steely strength was tempered by gentleness and wisdom, and she met my main criterion: she related to Jesse as a baby first, a baby with a seizure disorder second. And Dr. Spears was unafraid to try alternative treatments. On our first visit, she magically erased Jesse's teething pain by placing acupressure balls in his tiny ears. However, she, like everybody else, was unable to do anything about the seizure disorder. Her retirement returned us to the generic offices and the social dysfunction of generic neurologists who didn't seem to see our son.

When we moved to Massachusetts we again found grace, this time at Boston Children's Hospital. Dr. Sandy Helmers was a young, slim woman with hair the same color as her name. By then, our opening family act was unvarying; I picture us advancing into the random neurologist's office like a Roman phalanx, shields raised, with Jesse at the protected center. I would watch for any sign of empathy from each new doctor during our long recitation of Jesse's medical struggles and cognitive triumphs. If even a glimmer of warmth appeared, the shields went down and Jesse was revealed to the neurologist, Chris and I still hovering close by. Dr. Helmers looked directly at Jesse, asked him questions, reassured him.

She left for a position in Atlanta after only a couple of years. Her replacement was Dr. Elizabeth Thiele. By then we had become less wary that a neurologist would not see Jesse as sentient. Jesse was communicating well using his computer and was undeniably present in the world. He was enjoying school and doing well.

Still, some neurologists did not think about what the drugs they proposed would do to Jesse's alertness, his ability to think, to learn. They did not consider how blunting Jesse's learning would take away his greatest pride and pleasure. And so they proposed what was new on the market—wantonly, it felt to me. Each new course of drugs meant waiting and watching for the ever-present side effects, a full-court Internet study by me, and the usual outcome—no change. So the new shields went up, this time about drugs.

When I met Dr. Thiele, I asked her what new drug she would be pushing. She was my age, with a warm, open face. She laughed merrily and told me she was "much more granola than that." Then she concentrated on Jesse, cracking wise with him and making him grin. When she heard he wrote poetry, she asked Jesse if he would like to include one of his poems in an exhibition she was putting together of works by kids with epilepsy. I put down my shield and accepted grace when it fell upon all of us.

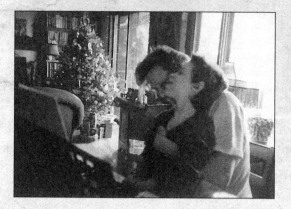

Chris and Jesse, age nine

My

Chair

Bumps

Through

The woods

As we look for

The perfect tree

We leave a piece of

Silver for the wood sprites

The decorations are in storage

We dust off all the ornaments

Dad spends an entire day stringing

Together popcorn and cranberries

I'm happy to have Dad home this Christmas

The tree's spine is crooked like mine and Mom's

Stan's homemade ornaments are placed on the tree

They hang on the branches like rings on fingers

Colored lights beat out white lights this year

This is our Charlie Brown Blue Spruce Christmas Tree

—Jesse's Christmas poem, 1999

CHAPTER SEVENTEEN

Collaboration

Jesse and I sat on the deck of our new house, a month after we moved, savoring summer heat that came with an ocean breeze as consistent as if someone flipped a daily switch across the tidal river. We were thrilled and still disconcerted to watch sailboats in our backyard, incongruously close to the highway—a reminder of our recent urban setting that was also visible from our deck. Chris joined us, his hands carefully cupped.

"Okay, Jesse. Wanna see something great? Open his hand, baby."

I stretched out Jesse's always-fisted hand in mine and Chris carefully placed a frog in it. Jesse shrieked with delight.

These were the homey joys of our first summer in a small New England town already imbued with my own happy childhood memories. For Jess it was frogs; for me, not having to drive around for forty-five minutes before squeezing my car into a shoebox-size parking space. Chris connected with his inner handyman.

Our next-door neighbors introduced themselves on the first day we moved in. Karen appeared at the door with homemade blueberry jam and her three children—Matthew, nine; Heather, eight; and Sarah, four—who came bearing handwritten welcome cards. Karen's husband, John, was an avid sailor, and took all of us on an exciting sail down the tidal river behind our homes and out into the bay beyond. After seventeen years of living in New York City and Hoboken, I was a little taken aback. There was no irony here, just warmth and an offer of friendship born of proximity.

Jesse and Sarah became constant companions and all four kids spent many snow days that winter snuggled on the sofa, watching movies and eating brownies, Jesse propped by strategically placed pillows. Sarah, a few years younger than Jess, was transfixed by the Greek myths I read to them. Her favorite was Persephone, the stolen bride of Hades, and Jess's was Perseus, the warrior who slew the sea monster to save Andromeda. When Jesse was a knight for Halloween a few years later, Sarah was his lady. They remained friends as they traversed the pimply shoals of adolescence, Sarah bopping in and out of our house and joining us for walks and annoying games of Marco Polo in the pool, Chris holding a suddenly lightweight Jesse under his arms, Jesse yelling incoherently and with gusto his own approximation of "Polo."

Chris and I hurtled headlong into small-town life, going to the pumpkin farm so Jesse could pick out his own jack-o'-

lantern, dressing up and going door-to-door for Halloween, caroling at the luminaries, an outdoor Christmas celebration with hayrides and free hot cider from the firehouse, and attending town meetings where votes were decided by a hand raised for "yea" or "nay."

We bought a bright red jogging stroller and marveled that for once we didn't wish we had engineering degrees from MIT so we could redesign it for Jesse's disability. This one worked just fine with the addition of pillows on either side of his head, and we crunched happily through the snowy woods collecting holly and fir boughs and picking out a Christmas tree. We usually traveled to my mother's house for the holidays, but on this first Christmas in our new home, we couldn't wait for Jesse to wake up in his own bed and not at Grandma's house thirty miles away.

On Christmas morning, Jesse couldn't spring from his bed, racing to see what Santa had left for him under that tree. A shard of sorrow pierced the day. But then I remembered my own puppylike eagerness on Christmas morning and my crushed disappointment over getting the doll instead of the book, or receiving the wrong-color sweater, and realized that it shouldn't be about what was under the tree. And for Jesse, it wasn't. He got presents all year round, the happy result of my yard sale travels on Saturday mornings with my old friend Maureen.

For Jesse, the magic happened later in the day, when the open house got under way and the living room pulsed with people and music and the savory smells of traditional food and a crackling fire. That's when Jesse's face would be alight with the wonder of the season. And that glow is the reward for every weary, overworked parent who climbs aboard the Polar Express year after year, that look of comfort and joy that graces a child's expression on Christmas day.

But school was the reason for the country-living experiment, and would be its testing ground. Jesse was placed in a classroom in a collaborative school program in a nearby town. Collaboratives in Massachusetts are put together from multiple school districts to share the cost of providing education to special-needs students. Because I was still relatively clueless about the meaning of full inclusion for children with disabilities, I was happy for the scraps that were offered to us at first.

Jesse was placed in a segregated classroom populated by disabled children, a special-needs teacher, and occupational, speech, and physical therapists. Suzanne was to be his personal aide—a nonnegotiable point on our side. The other kids in the class did not have one-on-one aides. We were also able to negotiate time for Jesse to spend daily in the regular first-grade classroom, but the bulk of his time was to be spent in the segregated classroom. We were grateful for the opportunity to figuratively dip our toes into inclusion because we thought the time spent in the regular first grade would be increased as time went on, slowly acclimating Jesse to being included in a regular classroom all day, every day. How, exactly, the time would be increased was not spelled out, but we thought we could work that out later. Our hope was based on our ignorance.

On the first day of school, Jesse was excited. He'd had a great summer swimming in the pool, going for walks in the woods and on nearby Duxbury beach, petting the animals at the Marshfield fair. But the real adventure would be the new school, meeting new kids, learning new things. By the time we got him into our new green van, he was giddy with anticipation. But soon after we arrived at the collaborative that was housed in a regular elementary school, after we walked past the smiles and greetings of his new principal, we reached his classroom. There we saw a message as clear as if it were a sign spanning the entry: you, Jesse Cooper, are disabled; therefore you are a second-class citizen.

Jesse's small "classroom" was at the very back of the school, an afterthought storeroom with no windows. All the other classrooms in this modern school, the ones for the normals, had windows looking out on trees and grass and sun. In Jesse's cramped place of learning, huge stinking blue gym mats used for the high school wrestling team were stored against the walls. Jesse's classmates were all severely physically disabled like him, but cognitively, they were on every point of the spectrum. There was a little girl who was paraplegic but verbally and mentally intact, alongside a little boy in a wheelchair with limited learning abilities. His only intellectual diversion was a balloon tied to his wheelchair, which the therapists urged him to hit.

When I left Jesse in that smelly room it felt like I was abandoning him to an institution. I felt ashamed, as if I had let a stranger walk up and spit on my child. I was devastated. Why did we move here? At least his segregated class in Hoboken had windows.

In my first-grade class we had one boy in leg braces from polio, a beautiful cherub with platinum curls who got around on crutches but, unlike Jesse, was verbal. He disappeared from my class at the end of the year. I felt relieved when he was gone. He scared me, somehow, and I could sense the hesitancy of the nuns when they were around him. Some of my other little friends were scared, too, though we never voiced the fear to each other. But we avoided him. The nun never took the time to explain to us that difference wasn't to be feared.

Years later, I caught up with him and he told me that he had stayed in school until the eighth grade, in another class, and that his school experience had been on the whole a good one. He had friends, played with kids in the neighborhood, and was included in their games. But in Sister Juventius's class, I only perceived that he was different, and then he was gone. That was the lesson I learned in first grade: Different = shun. Different = gone. I wanted to change that equation for Jesse.

When I think about Jesse's early education, I realize that it wasn't Jesse who had the slow learning curve. It was me. I was ignorant about how to make inclusion work. It took me forever, it seems, to figure out how Jesse could go to school in a community of peers, both disabled and nondisabled, and learn alongside them.

But the most important thing I learned from that first year at the collaborative was that Jesse would not necessarily be learning at school. His teachers and therapists were kind, responsible women with low expectations for Jesse. Because he was nonverbal, they provided a home/school book that listed what happened that day at school. We were to write back with questions or descriptions of Jesse's time at home and information about his health, moods, and upcoming doctor's appointments.

Before we could even consider the question of Jesse's

learning, I became obsessed with the stinking gym mats. By the end of the first week at school, I was in the principal's office demanding that they be removed.

That scenario followed a script I had enacted a few times by then, playing a stock character (Enraged Mother) with the medical profession and in the world of education. The generic plotline goes like this: I enter the office trying unsuccessfully to hide my quivering outrage. The Person in Charge, usually a man, asks me to sit down. I remain standing. I state my case in clipped sentences that sometimes get away from me, revealing the outrage I am trying to mask with professional tones. After I make a list of demands, a figurative Plexiglas shield comes down from the ceiling in front of the Person in Charge, who assumes a smooth professional demeanor meant to reassure the crazy lady opposite him. The Person in Charge smiles, takes notes, does nothing.

For two months, Jesse's home/school book resonated with escalating threats. I wrote in the book, "Hope mats are gone— otherwise R. [the principal] is DEAD MEAT." The mats were finally removed.

It took much longer to raise the school's expectations for Jesse. Around midyear, I finally got his teachers to agree to challenge him.

Home/School Book, 2/10/95

I was delighted to hear that Jesse finally showed you guys a little of what he knows. That's great. Actually, when I spell with him, I don't tell him how to spell the word, I usually just put two letters on one side [of his magnetic board], like A-R, and a few letters on the other side, like C, B, or J, and ask him "what makes that word CAR or JAR or BAR?" That way he figures it out for himself.

It took six months to get the teachers to let him spell out words instead of spelling out the words for him.

The speech therapist at the school had no expectations for Jesse at all. Let's call her Madame. She was French and upon my first meeting with her, she gargled at me with such a slushy accent that I regarded her with the incredulity of Alice meeting the hookah-smoking caterpillar.

At this point you may be wondering why a school system would hire a speech therapist with an accent thick as vichyssoise. You are now journeying with me through the looking glass of special education. The answer to your question is "Jam tomorrow, jam yesterday, but never jam today."

With all the gravitas of the Red Queen, Madame pronounced Jesse blind, and her written report said he couldn't "visually direct his gaze." (The following year, Jesse defeated his dad in a video game using his eyes to move the cursor on the eye-gaze computer at Boston College Campus School.) It was obvious that Madame also considered Jesse mentally challenged. No wonder: I don't think he ever understood a word she said.

I mercilessly mimicked her at home. In between feeding Jesse spoonfuls of beef stew during dinner, I pursed my lips and intoned, "Zzzhesee, Zzzhesee, *regardez-moi,* look at me, look at Madame." I struck an Edith Piaf pose by the oak table, my hands framing my face. "Ah, *mon petit chou,* am I not *jolie?* Direct your gaze to me, only me." My grand finale was to warble a few lines from "Non, je ne regrette rien." This impersonation never failed to make Jesse giggle. But it really wasn't funny. How could Jesse be helped by someone who firmly believed he was blind and mentally challenged? We decided to look elsewhere for speech therapy.

> *Home/School Book, 2/1/95*
> Jesse was videotaped at Duxbury Language and Learning Center. He responded beautifully to the therapist there and spelled "car," said "more" twice, said "hi," sailed through cognitive tests, visually directed his gaze and generally did more in two hours than in eight months of speech at school. Isn't that interesting?

Madame was tactful; she never addressed my entry in the home/school book, choosing instead to tell me about Jesse's "visit" that day to first grade, where Jesse's math work consisted of his reaching into a bucket and pulling out an object.

Jesse was receiving physical therapy at school, but we had also contracted a therapist named Holly shortly after we moved to Massachusetts, one who would do home visits. Holly was as clear as a stream, as elemental as rain, as good as bread. She was about my age, tall and lanky, with long straight hair, and her strong, gentle hands pulsed with heat when she worked on Jesse. The energy she radiated drew everyone in the house, including the dog. Goody clamored to be on the portable table she set up in the middle of our open dining/living space. He nestled happily in the crook of Jesse's arm and lay on his back for the entire session, paws in the air, basking in the spillover power Holly channeled to Jesse. Jesse was always relaxed and as supple as his tight limbs would allow after a session with Holly.

Holly was a registered physical therapist, but she also practiced craniosacral therapy, homeopathy, and Reiki. Over time, she treated the entire family, and appeared like a goddess of mercy for emergency sessions, when Jesse went into a dystonic state or once when I slipped on a rock in the woods and slammed my head so hard I couldn't feel my legs for a moment and thought Chris might be pushing two wheelchairs.

We also found a place for adaptive horseback riding, Handi-Kids, just a few towns over. Jess rode once a week. He loved the experience of being atop a huge beast and commanding it with his voice. His "clicks" told the horse—usually Sir Jay, an ancient lumbering dray horse—when to jolt Jesse forward along the outdoor track.

Jesse was having a very good school year. Everything was great—except for school. The "school" part of the home/school book usually read as a seizure log or a report on Jesse's moods of the day, happy or sad. When I read that he was chewing on his hands, I wrote back that Jesse was frustrated. I knew it was first grade (sort of) and quantum physics wasn't in the curriculum, but I also knew they were using flash cards to teach Jesse the alphabet, and he was chewing his hands because he already knew it. My frustration was growing along with Jesse's.

Holly once ran into Jesse's physical therapist from school and mentioned that she worked with him. The therapist rolled her eyes when Holly said my name—I was *that* mother, the one who thought her kid was bright, the one in deep denial about the extent of Jesse's disabilities.

Ultimately, no one involved with his education at the collaborative had any expectations for Jesse. Except Chris and me. I wanted Jesse to be in an actual first grade class, not a visitor to one. I wanted him to go to school in his own town with kids from his own neighborhood. I wanted him to learn what the other kids were learning. I wanted to remain "in denial."

The memory of that second autumn in our new home is lit by the sunny arrival of Brandy to our household and the hopeful anticipation of Jesse's coming school year in "real" first grade. It had been surprisingly easy to get the special ed director to agree to let Jesse start the year at our local elementary school, and we congratulated ourselves on making the choice to move to our little town. It took only a few months for Jesse to be pulled from "real" first grade and for us to learn about "dumping" and the art of war.

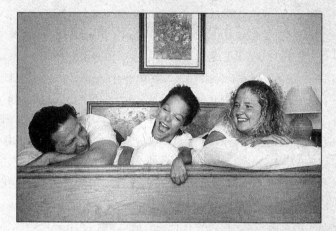

Jess, age ten, between Chris and Brandy in Montana

"I love you"

—*Jesse's actual words to Brandy, more than once*

CHAPTER EIGHTEEN

Brandy, You're a Fine Girl

W hen I think of Brandy, a series of photographs come to mind. My favorite is the one on the roof of the Le Montrose Suite Hotel in Los Angeles. Eight-year-old Jesse and twenty-two-year-old Brandy are wrapped in white terry-cloth hotel bathrobes, both wearing sunglasses, both lounging on a chaise by the pool, taking in the sun, Jess looking for all the world like a tiny Mafia don next to his chorus girl babe. And Brandy was a babe, make no mistake. Just twenty when she started her job with us, with blond ringlets that fell below her shoulders, crystal blue eyes, dazzling smile, and stacked, she was a rock star to Jesse's friends and a big sister and much more to our boy. And for us, there were the lobster perks! Brandy's lobsterman boyfriend, Dave, had grown up with the son of our dear friends Stan and Cathy. They were the ones who suggested that she'd be a great caregiver for Jess. Dave kept us supplied with lobsters and also venison when it was in season.

I see snapshots of Brandy smiling beside Jesse in his Halloween cowboy outfit, his wheelchair transformed into a fiery steed, or Jesse screaming with glee as Brandy races his chair away from a covey of geese chasing them in Montana. Snap: I see Brandy standing beside a transported Jesse with Xena, Warrior Princess—his womanly paradigm during his ten-year-old heroic phase—at Universal Theme Park. Snap: Brandy, smiling glassily, star-struck, holds Jesse as he swoons toward Jim Carrey (another idol), who was kind enough to share his lunch hour with us on the set of *Me, Myself & Irene.*

If you added a soundtrack to these visuals, you would hear the peals of laughter—Brandy's high-pitched giggle that spread like a flood tide under a full moon, and Jesse's ever-deepening, equally brimming chuckle, as the years with Brandy went by and he grew from boy to young man. Brandy defined fun, and added another dimension colored by her own youth. She remembered being a kid. She spoke kid, fluently. All of Jesse's friends were equally smitten.

When Jesse became an adolescent, it was Brandy who taught him grooming. They had facials together and she sent him to middle school every morning with his cowlicky fine hair spiked and gelled. (Kyle told me the first thing he noticed and envied about Jesse was his "cool hair.") Jesse and Brandy and his friends spent hours at the mall choosing scents at The Body Shop. Jesse settled finally on a body cream with the aroma of the woods we walked in every day. On some days now I go into his room and rub it on my hands, inhaling it like a drug that cracks the space-time continuum, taking me back to a moment when Jesse was the embodiment of that scent.

Brandy got to know Jesse on her first week with us via some dog vomit. Jess and Brandy were watching television while Chris and I were on a date night. Brandy got up for something and sat down heavily in the overstuffed green chair. Jess clicked his "kiss" sound urgently and inclined his head toward Brandy.

"What is it, Jesse? Are you thirsty?"

Another urgent click and head bob.

"You're thirsty."

A headshake. "No."

"You're not thirsty?"

Another click. Head bob.

"What is it? Okay, I'll get the computer."

Jess watched her intensely, holding his breath. Brandy put her hand down, stood up, looked down, and saw she had been sitting in a pool of Goody's vomit. Jesse laughed, delighted. A seven-year-old's dream come true! A Jim Carrey moment in his own living room! Brandy said those pure-kid moments just affirmed what she knew about him from the first day she met him: he was a kid first, disabled kid second. She "got" him.

Brandy was the yin to my yang in kid matters. I admit it, theme parks didn't do it for me. From Spooky Town to Universal to Edaville Railroad, I was always repelled by the forced cheer of these places and turned into a muttering old coot the minute I crossed the entrance booth. Brandy loved them and so did Jess. Everyone was happy when she assumed the duties of theme park guide. Chris liked Universal, and took Jess on all the daredevil rides, but he also liked bringing snakes and frogs into the house so Jess could hold them in his hand. Brandy and I always provided added sideline excitement, going into high girly mode at the sight of slimy things, emitting little squeaks and cries of disgust, and uniting Chris and Jess in manly solidarity.

Brandy was with us through hard times, too. The first time Jesse had an attack of dystonia, when he was eight, we didn't know what it was. We were frightened out of our minds; dystonia can look like a seizure that has no end. Jesse's muscles contracted over and over as his whole body twisted and jerked in painful, unending spasms. He seemed insensate, unable to communicate. We rushed to Children's Hospital in Boston in a state of sheer terror, me driving frenziedly, Brandy cradling Jesse's writhing body in the backseat. I called Chris in Florida and he made plans to leave the set of the film he was shooting and join us as soon as he could get a flight.

When we got to the emergency room we couldn't reach our neurologist, Dr. Helmers, and young interns who didn't look old enough to babysit Jesse were conferring outside our cubicle. The room was spinning. I sat on the gurney with Jess, trying not to faint. Someone came in to take a blood sample from Jess and it sprayed all over Brandy. I demanded to know what the interns were saying and they excitedly told me they might have to take a brain biopsy. I told them they would do nothing of the sort.

I always think of my mother in situations like that and am grateful that I speak English. Jesse's diagnosis was turning into an experimental free-for-all, with a brigade of doctors asking me if possibly I had migraines because maybe that's what this was. I did have migraines in the past, I told them, before I cured them with evening primrose oil. They were like boy detectives on a sugar high. Maybe there was a genetic quotient! Maybe this was a migraine! If so, they could shoot Jesse up with a new miracle drug and the migraine would be gone, instantly.

Really? This didn't look like any migraine I ever had.

I realized with a sinking heart that none of the doctors knew what was going on. I told Brandy she should take the subway into Boston, and then take the bus home. It looked like it would be a long night. She looked at me, horrified.

"I can't take the subway!"

I realized that Brandy, a small-town girl, was more afraid of taking the subway than staying in this hellhole.

"Don't worry, Brandy, you're covered in blood. You look insane, no one will come near you," I told her.

We looked at each other. No words, just giggles that were really high-pitched shrieks, the prelude to hysteria. She stayed. Chris arrived. Jesse suffered for three days without a diagnosis before the attack finally ended. Now we were bonded in blood: Jesse, Brandy, Chris, and me.

The diagnosis of dystonia would only come *four years later,* during another frightening attack in Los Angeles. Dr. Thiele diagnosed it correctly—over the phone.

Brandy became our daughter. Our family was like a weird hippie cult to her, one she couldn't wait to join. She had had a bare-bones childhood, raised by a single mom, money always tight, divorced dad far away in California and rarely seen. Brandy was putting dinner on the table at thirteen. She wistfully said to me one day, "So, when you came home from school, like, your mother was *there*, right?"

I wanted to cry. Brandy gave so much care and love and pampering to Jesse and she hadn't had much of it herself growing up. Brandy was like a girl in a fairy tale; she had retained an essential innocence in her core, along with the curiosity and guilelessness of a child. That was her bridge to Jesse, and the reason he loved her with all his heart.

Oh, the pleasure of mentoring a young woman who wants to learn! Brandy, like Jesse, was hungry for words. We read Yeats, Wordsworth, Whitman. We all loved the drama of opera, screaming along with the high sopranos as we baked cookies, the volume set dangerously high, Brandy guiding Jesse's hand to crack an egg in perfect tandem with our eardrums splintering. As an encore, we'd stir and jiggle to "Born to Run," Jesse yelling "Bruuuuuu!"

Brandy and I boarded countless planes together, a two-woman SWAT team whizzing Jesse through security and settling him into his seat. She was also a member of the grizzly pack of Jesse protectors from day one.

Both she and Jesse were crazed with excitement on the occasion of their first Hollywood premiere, the opening of *Seabiscuit*, in which Chris had a supporting role as the horse trainer. Their limo followed ours and kept circling as Chris and I walked the red carpet.

Once they parked, the circling and delirium got to Jesse and he vomited all over his carefully chosen outfit for the premiere. Brandy was stuck in the parking lot behind the theater with Jesse crying, upset, and covered with vomit. Cara Tripicchio,

Chris's caring and super-efficient publicist, pulled me off the line and told me what happened. I gave her a hundred dollars and asked her to go to the nearby Gap and get him a T-shirt and jeans. Meanwhile, I headed over to the parking lot, just in time to see the paparazzi advancing on the limo. We were furious. Brandy shielded Jesse with her body, I alerted Cara's publicists, and a mini-army of harpy publicists descended on the paparazzi, backing them off. Cara returned with the outfit and all was well. Except that later I asked her if there was change from the hundred I had given her. It turned out Jesse's little black track suit cost a hundred thirty dollars, about four times what I had shelled out for the thrift shop dress I had worn.

When Chris filmed *My House in Umbria,* we spent a glorious month at a villa in Tuscany, teenage Jesse lounging by the pool surrounded by vineyards, Brandy squealing as the occasional lizard ran across her legs. We all sat in the cool marble of the Duomo in Florence, where Brandy burst into tears. I told her about the Italian word *Stendhalismo,* which describes being overcome by the harmony and beauty of all things around you, because Stendhal, a nineteenth-century French writer, had become short of breath, heart racing, near fainting at the art and beauty surrounding him in Florence. That's how it worked with our family now that Brandy was with us. *Stendhalismo,* almost all the time.

■

The last snapshot: Brandy writhes, wailing, her face buried in Jesse's sheets, fingers raking the covers over and over, moments after I have told her that Jesse is gone from us. She is delirious; she searches for flesh, smells, a connection. I stand watching her from far away, in a place of hollow calm, at the epicenter of grief. She is a physical mirror of my own utter devastation.

Right before Christmas, two years after Jesse's death, we sit with Brandy at our scarred oak table and pour the wine after sharing dinner. She now lives far away, in upstate New York, and a visit is a rare treat. Brandy praises the meal, but what she gives us in return is priceless: a perfectly formed memory of a moment in time with Jesse. She hands Chris a framed picture: Brandy, Jesse, Chris, all laughing, lying prone on a hotel bed in Montana. Brandy reminds us they were watching *Willie Wonka and the Chocolate Factory* and that the Oompa Loompas, the little orange-skinned men in the movie, made them all laugh, Jesse most of all. In the picture, Jesse is in the center, and Chris and Brandy are on either side, looking at him, a reminder that all of us had for a brief moment in time Jesse at the center of our lives.

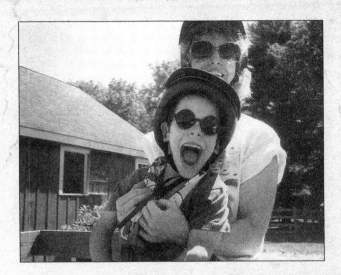

Jess, seven, riding Sir Jay at Handi-Kids

"There is a young cowboy, he lives on the range . . ."
—*"Sweet Baby James" by James Taylor*

CHAPTER NINETEEN
Bad Behavior

This is about guilt. Corrosive, molten-lava guilt that puts your soul in the burn unit. And this is about forgiving yourself, and what it takes to become a mother from hell.

I am sitting at my kitchen desk, reading Jesse's home/school book from his first few months of inclusion in the first grade of our local elementary school. Brandy has pasted a laughing picture of Jesse riding Sir Jay on the cover of the battered blue notebook. The notebook should have been a means for parent, aide, and teacher to report the daily events at school of a child who doesn't communicate in the usual way. Instead it reads like a cryptogram, and it soon becomes clear that I was unaware of the code.

I don't even recognize myself, this perky yet cringing poseur trying to stay upbeat on the home pages of the home/

school book as Jesse's school year unwinds toward an inevitable implosion. When I ask myself now, fourteen years later, how I missed the signs, I still don't have an answer.

Home/School Book, September 1995
Jesse had a great first day! ☺
—*Jesse's teacher*

Jesse had a great night!
—*Jesse's mother*

It went steeply downhill from there.

Jesse's teacher was in her early twenties—tall, willowy, baby-faced and baby-voiced, and very, very sure of herself. She was convinced of the rightness of everything she had read in her textbooks about how to run her classroom and was eager to put her newfound knowledge into practice. She had volunteered to accept Jesse into her first-grade classroom, and I was happy that she wanted him. Jesse was assigned an aide, a large middle-aged blonde who was also the mother of three children. The aide was to give Jesse snacks and lunch, assist him in the classroom, and deliver him to the occupational and speech therapists, who worked with him in a separate location. Jesse was the only child in the elementary school in a wheelchair, the only nonverbal child, the only child with severe disabilities.

According to Jesse's teacher, there was appropriate behavior and inappropriate behavior for first grade, and Jesse's behavior was mostly inappropriate. He cried. A lot. He cried when the aide tried to make him hold a crayon and draw pictures. He cried when he bit his tongue and drew blood. He cried when he was constipated. He cried when the aide left his leg braces on for three hours, when the limit was twenty minutes—after which the braces, which were made of unyielding plastic and encased Jesse's legs up to his knees, would leave welts. And they were hot. No wonder they made him cry. But the crying was disruptive to the rest of the class, Jesse's teacher informed me in her rounded cursive. They were going to throw him out. He would be evicted for crying.

God, please let them want to teach my child. Please make him stop crying. What if they don't let him stay in school? These fears triumphed over the overprotective mother who had managed to keep Jesse safe this far into his educational career. But I never wrote about these fears to Jesse's teacher when I responded in the home/school book. Even my handwriting looks different on those pages. My usual script is a series of hurried jagged peaks and contrasting generous loops, but that's when I am myself, not someone cowed by authority. In the home/ school book I used my old Catholic schoolgirl penmanship, as if my persona had reverted back to those years when I was told what to do at school and kept my head down to avoid trouble, like a broken prisoner of war.

I was glad at least that he hadn't used the aide as his Bitey Boy. He had been known to bite when he was furiously angry and had even bitten me once. I put him in his room for a time-out and told him he was staying there until he apologized. He could call me when he was ready. He yelled for me after about ten minutes, and when I asked Jesse if he was sorry, he clicked "yes." If I were furious and seven years old and couldn't stomp around, throw things, mouth off, or run in circles, I would probably bite, too. But I couldn't let my compassion get in the way and help raise a severely disabled spoiled brat. I told Jesse firmly that biting was forbidden, that there would be consequences and that I never wanted to see that happen again. It didn't, but the crying at school continued. He cried so much that he came home miserable, his face tear-streaked, his clothes damp and sweaty.

Jesse's teacher said that the crying was "behavior." She said that he was manipulating all of us, that he didn't want to be at school. She said he stopped crying whenever she or the aide said the word *home,* because at home he was allowed to do whatever he wished.

Home/School Book, October 1995

I'm sorry for being so blunt but this behavior for any reason at seven years old is unacceptable. We do not allow it with the other kids and it will not be allowed [for] Jesse. He is very smart and is capable of showing his needs, or emotions in another way, even if it his physical [sic].

—*Jesse's teacher*

Very touchy about front tooth—it bled—he freaked last night. Hope he's better today.

P.S. You guys are terrific—I think you'll be a real force for positive change in Jesse's life.

—*Jesse's Appeaser Mother*

"I think you'll be a real force for positive change in Jesse's life." I had to hack phragmites in the marsh for two hours after rereading that cowardly piece of pandering. I stood in the center of the ten-foot reeds, unable to see. I wanted to be lost, to lose myself in the repetitive motions of cutting, stomping, yanking the fucking stupid stalks out by the roots. I worked mechanically, muttering "stupid, stupid, stupid," as I tried to burn off the shameful memories of my own complicity and ignorance. I worked until my body was as twisted as Jesse's little fingers were when the aide stuffed them hurriedly into his coat sleeve at the end of a day at school.

> *Home/School Book, October, 1995*
> Jesse definately [sic] wasn't upset over his tooth yesterday. He ate snack and was fine after snack. It started when [the aide] asked him to write. I know it is hard to break the pattern of looking for something physical and not emotional. Yesterday was definately [sic] emotional, and behavioral. Jesse is used to not doing things he doesn't want to. He had a good morning. In the afternoon Jesse had to leave the room. He started screaming as soon as he was asked to color the life of a pumpkin book.
> —*Jesse's teacher*

Maybe Jesse was just prescient. Maybe he knew he wouldn't be holding a crayon or a pen in the future. Maybe he knew he would be using his raking grasp for a pull switch on a computer in second grade instead of writing with a pen.

It didn't matter. We sided with his teacher. We punished Jesse. We took away his horseback riding. On days he cried so hard we had to come to school and get him, we punished him by putting him in his room and closing the door. We condoned the idiocy of the crayon he had no way of using.

Even though we knew he was already reading sentences, and Jesse's teacher's class was still learning the alphabet, we didn't dare bring up that he might in fact be bored. We believed his teacher: that he was being manipulative, that he didn't want to work, that we had to break the pattern of Jesse "not doing things he doesn't want to."

We appeased, collaborated, and I continued to write cheerleadery rah-rah responses to Jesse's teacher's misspelled messages.

Jesse didn't always feel well. He had seizures. His bowels were so irregular we took him to a holistic doctor who ran a series of tests to see if he was vitamin deficient. The spasticity that tightened his limbs also affected his colon; we were very careful to give Jesse foods that helped him eliminate because I had read that constipation could increase seizure activity. He was always hungry. Jesse's teacher accepted none of these physical realities as reasons for his behavior. She suspected mutiny, and mutiny was not to be allowed in her very first classroom.

Chris was away a lot in September and October filming in New York. We talked every day, but they were often fourteen-hour days for him and while I duly reported the mostly bad news from school, there was little he could do from a movie set except commiserate and promise to be home soon. He was shooting an action film and I really didn't want him preoccupied while he zigzagged through New York traffic, playing a murderer trying to escape his pursuers. He would be home for the holidays. I could hold out until then. I wrote to Jesse's teacher begging her to please first consider eliminating any physical reason before she came to the conclusion that he was exhibiting "behavior."

By November, I began to doubt the "Jesse is a little rebel" theory. Jesse never threw tantrums at home. We had seen frustration over miscommunication, and crankiness over an upset stomach or constipation, but his temperament was generally sunny.

Home/School Book, November, 1995
But to be honest Marianne I am and [the aide] is getting very discouraged and not because of Jesse's behavior. We are discouraged because everytime [sic] we tell you Jesse is having a behavior it seems there is a reason for it. A stomache [sic], cold, seizure, etc. Marianne until you realize and Chris realize this behavior is not acceptable for any reason [sic].
It is not even acceptable for pain.
—*Jesse's teacher*

"It is not even acceptable for pain."

That sentence roused me from slumber, and the mother bear came out of hibernation.

The fantasy of full inclusion for Jesse poofed into a dust bunny that rolled under my desk, the same one where I (or someone impersonating me) wrote effusive messages of praise in the home/school book. Full inclusion wasn't going to happen with this clueless teacher. It wasn't going to happen by making Jesse hold a crayon and draw pumpkins. But I didn't know yet how to make it happen. I only knew that the cheerleader who wrote those messages was gone, and the seething mother from hell was ascendant. This mother fantasized about Jesse's childless teacher shaking her colicky newborn, shouting, "Stop crying! This isn't appropriate!" or telling her screaming, bleeding five-year-old in the emergency room, "This is not acceptable! *It is not even acceptable for pain!*"

Full disclosure: I didn't just fantasize the colicky baby. I wished it on Jesse's teacher like a witch in a fairy tale: everlasting days and nights of sleep-destroying, madness-inducing, nonstop crying with no end in sight.

To Jesse's teacher, I actually said nothing. But I didn't lumber back into my cave. I rose up, sniffing the air, suddenly alert.

Jesse still had good days at school, days when the aide would deliver him to me at the end of the day and I covered him with kisses, relieved that I was picking him up at the usual time and that he wasn't trembling and wet with tears before lunch. He made friends, too, Adam and Kelham, neither one the sensitive type you'd think would be attracted to a nonverbal kid in a wheelchair.

Adam told his mother there was a kid in his class who hated to color as much as he did, and could they have him over to visit? A few weeks later he asked his mom, "What does nonverbal mean?" His mother told him. Adam was puzzled: "But Jesse can talk, people just don't listen." Adam's mom, Lynne, was shocked when she met Jesse. Adam hadn't mentioned the wheelchair. It just wasn't important to him as the mutual hatred of coloring was. When Jesse came over to visit, Adam and his brother, Derek, included him in their boisterous games, Jesse shrieking with laughter as they maneuvered his wheelchair in a dizzying game of tag. I sipped coffee with Lynne, trying not to bolt from my chair and wrest away the wheelchair. Later they became bowling buddies one day a week at the local lanes, Jesse pushing the ball down a chute that fitted over his chair, Adam carefully positioning the chute. Their team was called the Outlaws.

I met Kelham's mother, Jo, at a Thanksgiving party for first graders. We gravitated toward one another, the only mothers in the place not wearing themed sweaters, the only mothers in black. We next met at a local store, where Jo told me she had been in class to help out and in her opinion Jesse was bored. They had been working on colors yet again, and Jesse was put on her knee for her to "look after him." He began to squirm and Jo told the teacher he needed the bathroom. No one listened, according to Jo. "Nor did they ever," she says now.

Kelham was British and gifted; he bonded with Jesse because they were both bored and got into trouble a lot at school. Jesse's teacher recommended holding Kelham back "on social grounds," but when he pushed Jesse in his wheelchair, he told me he had to practice because he "might have a wife in a wheelchair some day." One day I heard him read aloud in class; he was more adept than Jesse's teacher and stumbled less over the words in the text. I wondered who should be held back.

Despite the intermittent good reports from school, there were little darts of doom, such as when my neighbor Karen voiced her concern over the way she had seen the aide feeding Jesse in the cafeteria during lunch. "Marianne, she had one hand on his forehead and his head was tipped back and she wasn't giving him time to breathe between bites." Even though that image reverberated in my brain during sleepless nights, I said nothing. I said nothing to Jesse's teacher. And I sent him back to school, where he was unhappy almost every day.

I didn't know how to help them teach Jesse. I thought they would know what to do. I thought they would have his best interests at heart. I was slow to understand what I should have known from early intervention, from preschool, from kindergarten, from the collaborative—that we, Jesse's parents, must be the driving force behind his education and his greatest advocates. Years after the fact, I still feel like I should be paraded through the streets of our small town, barefoot, my head shaven, like a traitor who collaborated with the enemy and betrayed not only her country but her own seven-year-old son.

I called Mary Somoza in New York and told her it wasn't working. On her recommendation, I began to keep a list in a notebook of my own, a careful record of every time I called the school and received no answer, all correspondence to and from the school, in preparation for future mediations or even a lawsuit. Mary explained to me what "dumping" was, and how to advocate for your child's civil rights.

Dumping is a setup for failure. It's when the school accedes to the parents' wish to include their child in a regular classroom, but does so without any supports in place—which guarantees the program's failure. It's placing a severely physically disabled child in a regular classroom without a special education teacher there to modify the curriculum. In first grade, when students are coloring with crayons, inclusion means finding an alternative method for a quadriplegic child to do a similar activity like finger-painting or using a drawing program on a computer. Inclusion means making sure the one-on-one aide assigned to that child can facilitate communication for a non-verbal child via computer or message board.

I was realizing that full inclusion would never happen magically, on its own. I would have to make it happen.

Jesse was having tantrums again in January after Christmas vacation. We asked Brandy to go into school one morning and observe. When I arrived at the school to pick her up, she was standing stiffly on the curb with a smile that looked wobbly and wrong on her face. Her blue eyes were huge and glassy. Back at the house, the story unfolded slowly, every word a dagger thrust. In tears, Brandy said that the aide thought Brandy hated her job as much as the aide did. While in the classroom, the aide complained about my picking Jesse up at the end of the day and "kissing him all over with that red lipstick of hers, right in front of the fifth and sixth graders." Brandy said she spoke over Jesse's head in the middle of the classroom about how "he don't belong here," and "between you and me, Brandy, we both know where he's gonna end up." Jesse yelled his objections throughout her speech, and was told to "be quiet." Then Jesse's teacher chimed in about me, her Betty Boop voice an excited near-whisper: "She really needs to learn to let go; we don't know the life expectancy of a CP kid." She talked about my child dying in front of him. I pictured Jesse listening, frightened. I saw myself towering over the teacher, my Medusa self

unleashed, snaky hair standing on end, shrieking a curse that
would send her to hell.

Chris sat at the table, deceptively still. Then he abruptly
picked Jesse up and lay with him on Jesse's bed, cradling him,
crooning. I walked to the phone in a trance of fury and called
the principal. I wanted a meeting now—this minute, this very
second—so I could confront them all. The aide. The teacher.
The special ed director, too. He was the one who had set up
this scenario. Did he plan this debacle from the beginning?
Was he aided and abetted by the inexperienced teacher and
the casually cruel aide? Did he hope that by dumping Jesse, the
program would fail and we'd go away?

It was Friday. The principal arranged a meeting for the following Monday. I didn't know if I could wait until then. In the
last few minutes I had joined the berserker tribe of mothers,
those who go into battle without any armor but rage. Mad as
dogs, fierce as wolves, they fight to the death.

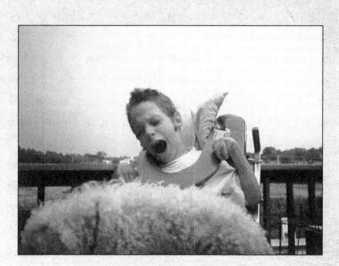

Jess, ten, enraged on our deck

CHAPTER TWENTY

Rageaholic

I'm a rageaholic. This is how it's always been: I black out momentarily and wake to find myself lunging at someone. I speak in tongues of flame. Spittle-flecked venom showers everywhere, like a fireworks display gone horribly wrong. Onlookers ooh and ahh in horror instead of wonder. The intelligible speech part of my brain shuts down with an audible click and I have no control over the sounds that spew forth. The sounds are part animal, part human, with occasional recognizable words. A flush begins in my chest, crawls up my throat, ends at my hairline. I wear the mask of red rage.

I wonder if someday I'll find an inert body at my feet when I am sane again, seconds after. Could I kill someone in a moment of fury? Afterward, I wonder about the gibberish I screeched. I muse about how I looked, like a nightmare creature crouched atop a flying buttress. I'm ashamed. There is a comical element to my rage; I look ridiculous, like a toddler. I'm too short for a towering rage. I'm like Rumpelstiltskin. I feel afraid: this much rage isn't normal. I read up on spontaneous human combustion. I have dreams of being in prison for accidentally killing someone, in just such a moment.

In New York City, I have to outrun a crazy man after I pound on his car, Ratso Rizzo–style, for cutting me off when I cross the street. Then, a blackout rage happens during an acting exercise. Suddenly I'm screaming my response and I don't remember what I said.

I decide to go to a shrink. I tell the shrink I don't want to talk about my childhood. I only want to control the rage. But I think about my childhood anyway. I remember being four years old and walking home from kindergarten with pudgy, easygoing Alex and his mother. I remember how I turned around and slapped him across the face as hard as I could, with his mother standing there, right in front of Larry's Superette. I don't remember why I slapped him. I just remember being shocked at myself after I did it.

I am surprised when the shrink actually helps me control the rage. She doesn't give me drugs. She gives me "coping mechanisms." I learn not to ignore small irritants. I learn to speak up when the stakes are low, before the blackout rage comes. It works. It works for years.

It works until I have Jesse.

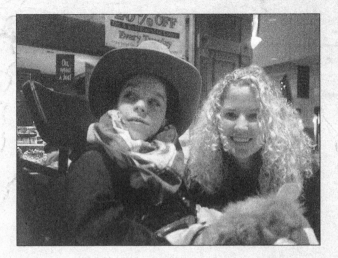

Jesse, eight, with Brandy on Halloween

Love.
Kind, wonderful;
Exciting, liberating, living;
Virtue, peace, grudge, lie;
Enraging, fighting, crying;
Ugly, horrible.
Hate.

—*Jesse Cooper*

CHAPTER TWENTY-ONE

How Do You Solve a Problem Like Maria?

"I just want them in tears by the end of this meeting. That's all I want," I told Chris. I had no long-term plans beyond a reckoning for Jesse, a public shaming of the clueless and cruel adults who made him cry at school. The night before the meeting I lay beside Jesse nose to nose and whispered my vows to him: he would never have to see that aide again; he would have a different teacher; and finally, he would return to school and learn as joyously there as he did at home. I had no idea how I would make all this happen.

We were crammed around a rectangular table in a box-like meeting room at Jesse's school. I sat directly across from Jesse's teacher and never took my eyes off her. She did not meet mine. The aide sat beside the teacher, her beefy arms folded defiantly. Brandy was tucked protectively between Chris and me. The principal, a large imposing man with a bullhorn voice, sat next to Chris, and beside me sat the special ed director, our very own speed bump on the zigzaggy road of Jesse's educational life.

I was ready for combat, a ninja mother with black leggings, a beret, and a fuck-you double slather of red lipstick—enough to drive Jesse's aide demented, I hoped.

A greatest-hits medley ran over and over in my mind, like a horrible, catchy jingle of hate.

"He don't belong here."

"She really needs to learn to let go. We don't know the life expectancy of a CP kid."

"We both know where he's gonna end up."

"Crying isn't acceptable. It's not even acceptable for pain."

Let's see you cry now, Jesse's teacher. Cry me a river, Jesse's aide. You were supposed to be helping him.

Jesse was at home watching cartoons with our neighbor Karen and little Sarah. He was safe, for now. But how long could we keep him home from school?

Our first meeting with the special ed director, more than a year earlier, had been friendly; there were smiles and handshakes, and he asked us to call him by his first name. That was when we agreed to put Jesse in the collaborative and made tentative noises about inclusion. After that, he graciously allowed Jesse to be a "visitor" in Miss LaGreca's first grade class. We weren't a problem then. We were now.

I didn't ever call him by his first name. Something in

me resisted that attempt at bonhomie, a sixth sense that we wouldn't actually be friends on a first-name basis, that the smiles masked a martinet's nature. At first he was Mr. Insert Generic Irish Catholic Surname Here. Later I knew him by an ever-changing roster of obscenities. Finally, after he mentioned at one meeting how much he admired the von Trapp family (caramelized forever in *The Sound of Music*), he became Maria von Trapp. In these pages, I'll just call him the sped director. He was slight of stature, only a few inches taller than me, with sharp features and small, darting eyes. At our first meeting, he wore a too small green blazer with his bony wrists protruding and the emblem of a Catholic college over his heart. I had an unpleasant flashback to Our Lady Help of Christians High School and the general aura of torment surrounding those years.

The sped director opened the meeting and Brandy nervously consulted her notes, reporting what she'd seen and heard in a quavering voice. There was silence. We all looked at Jesse's teacher. She began to cry. Good. Check one off the list.

"But I didn't mean it the way it sounded. Brandy's making it sound worse than it was!"

She was sorry, so sorry, she continued, in her baby-doll voice. I sat stonily, unmoved. Jesse's aide, on the other hand, denied everything.

"I didn't do nothin'."

She stared belligerently at Brandy, challenging her. Brandy made a shocked sound of disbelief, which the aide chose to interpret as a laugh.

"It's not funny, Brandy. It's nothin' to laugh about," smirked the aide in a concerned voice that didn't hide a triumphant underlying "gotcha."

So that's how it would be: kill the messenger. I took one look at Brandy's stricken face and had a rage blackout. I "came to" halfway across the table with my arms extended in a throttling position toward the aide's meaty neck. My own neck was mottled and red. I sputtered wordlessly in an ecstasy of rage. Chris half rose from his seat, reflexively, his own face bright red.

Before I had the satisfaction of physical contact, the nasal voice of the sped director cut through the berserker haze. "Okay, let's all calm down. We're a team here."

I sat back down and Brandy resumed her report, her voice even shakier now that violence was in the air. The sped director dismissed Brandy's input as if she were a ditzy blond bimbo wrapped sinuously around a pole instead of a serious young woman earnestly consulting her notes about Jesse's day in school.

We proposed that Jesse spend the rest of the year with the special education teacher, Maura, and a different aide, and that Brandy fill in for the aide in the interim. The situation was so dire that we were willing to regress back to segregation for the rest of the year and try again in second grade. The sped director agreed graciously to Jesse's being segregated with the special education teacher, which was what he had wanted all along.

He dismissed the idea of Brandy's becoming Jesse's aide, saying it was "inappropriate." I pointed out that her qualifications were better than Jesse's current aide (Brandy was a certified nurse's assistant) and that she had the advantage of knowing how to work with Jesse, since she did so at home. I also made it clear that Brandy would work as Jesse's aide at no cost to the school, since we were already paying her for a full day. The sped director spelled it out: we were to have no input as to the person who would be toileting, feeding, and helping to educate our son. The school chose the aide. Period.

I asked what qualifications were necessary to become an aide in the school system.

"A high school diploma and a good personality," he answered. "But the school chooses the aide."

"Okay, this is a waste of time. This is insane." I gathered my notes. Jesse with that aide? Unthinkable.

"Please sit down, Mrs. Cooper. The meeting isn't over." The sped director now proposed that we call in a "behavior expert" to deal with Jesse's crying. And that Jesse be tested by a neuropsychologist. And that we keep the same aide. The meeting adjourned with nothing decided about Jesse's immediate school future.

On the way home to Jesse, we were silent, stunned.

"He's not going back there. Not with her," I finally pronounced. Chris and I agreed we would keep Jesse home with us until we were sure he was safe. We arrived home to Jesse's expectant face, a sunflower. Brandy couldn't hide her tears. Chris swept Jesse into his arms and swung him around to make him giggle. I couldn't look at my boy and tell him he would be staying home from school. But he knew. Brandy's tears, his dad's forced jollity, and my set face told him. He knew. There would be no school on Monday.

All weekend the song lyrics to "How Do You Solve a Problem Like Maria" from *The Sound of Music* skipped through my head like a chorus of nuns on crack. Three days after the meeting I called the sped director. I went downstairs where Jesse couldn't hear me.

"Have you considered the proposal we brought up at the meeting?" I asked.

"What proposal?"

"The one where Jesse stays in Maura's class for the rest of the year with a new aide, preferably Brandy."

"She's not appropriate."

"What does 'appropriate' mean?"

"I didn't like the way she talked to me at that meeting."

That remark left me speechless. Brandy's shaky voice hadn't risen above a whisper in the meeting. And where was *Jesse* in this mix? *He,* the sped director, didn't like the way Brandy spoke to *him.* I tried to get the conversation back on track.

"What about the rest of the proposal?"

"I don't remember that proposal. His teacher apologized and we agreed to call in a behavior expert. That was the resolution."

"Jesse's not safe at school," I said. I paced around the basement, Jesse's hangout room, my eyes on the shelves filled with books and computer games.

"You should send Jesse to school."

"Or else what?"

"You should send him to school."

This time I heard clearly the threat. I was wearing a hole in the floor. "I'm calling a lawyer."

"I'll set a date for a meeting to discuss mediation," he said. On that bleak note, I hung up. Mediation could be the final step before an actual lawsuit.

This wasn't about Jesse, or his education. It felt like a power play by the sped director. We wanted input on the aide. The sped director insisted we keep the same aide who felt "Jesse don't belong here."

Now I knew who this guy was. The green blazer with the Catholic college emblazoned over his heart was the first clue. This power play made it all clear: he was the kid who always eagerly shot up his hand to tell the nun who talked while she was out of the room. He was the hall monitor who reported kids for the slightest infraction of the rules. He was the picked-on, wedgied, noogied little prig who knew without a doubt that he was going to heaven and I was going to hell. And now he was in a position to unleash a hell of his very own making on all of us.

Our disagreement wasn't about inclusion. It was about the wielding of power for the sake of power. It was payback for something that Jesse, the innocent victim in all of this, never did.

Calls to the superintendent, a mysterious Wizard-of-Oz-like character whom I could never get on the phone, went unanswered. He never came out from behind the curtain, not once, during the entire two-year battle with the school system over Jesse's future.

A call to the principal, who had remained mostly silent during the meeting with the sped director, got us a private audience with him the following week in his office. There Chris and I were told that he was angry with the sped director for not supporting inclusion, but not to repeat that outside the office, because he would deny he said it. The principal proposed a new IEP with "support" and another meeting of the "team," but he wouldn't budge on the aide. We were to have no input.

I was perplexed by the principal. He seemed sympathetic; I knew that he had disability in his family. In November, he had arranged for Jesse to participate in the eye-gaze computer program at Boston College. There Jesse was able to demonstrate to Maura that he could read. The aide was also along for that trip, but apparently Jesse's reading skills didn't change her mind about his "not belonging" in first grade at his local elementary school. Did the principal support inclusion or didn't he?

In the end, the principal's views on inclusion didn't matter—the aide was the deal breaker, for us and for them. The battle lines were drawn and neither side would budge: they didn't want a whistleblower and we didn't want that aide anywhere near our son. No one wanted to have their power threatened, not the sped director, nor the principal, even though the safety of our child was at stake.

The administration hoped we'd all just give up and go away.

At school, the principal told my friend Jo, Kelham's mom, "The Coopers have made other plans for Jesse." Jo told him we wanted Jess back at school, just with a different aide. He grew visibly angry with that. "I choose the aide. Next thing you'll have parents wanting to fire the principal."

We received notice of a twenty-dollar fine in the mail from the school for "disruption of services," the icing on the cake. The letter, signed by the principal, bombarded us with officialese, a new language we were learning the hard way. It said that we were being fined for keeping Jesse home from school. It felt as if we were being penalized for protecting our child.

Jesse was home every day. He saw his friends Kelham and Adam after school, but Brandy and I dreaded the mornings. Jesse often cried when he heard the school bus picking up our neighbors at the top of the drive. His tears were an acid drip, a slow and steady corrosion of my heart. We filled his days with books and music, trips to museums, and educational activities, but he wasn't learning with other kids. He was depressed.

Adam called the house about a week after Jesse had been home. "Why isn't Jesse in school?" he asked.

I tried to explain in a way that a seven-year-old might understand.

"You know how you learned about people of color not being allowed to go to school? Well, there are people at the school who think people in wheelchairs shouldn't be allowed to go to school."

Adam was outraged.

"But . . . that's just on the *outside!*"

Too bad the adults in the school hierarchy didn't think like seven-year-olds.

The lonely winter days went by. Jesse wasn't at school. He was isolated, sad, immured. I made more calls to the superintendent, always unanswered. I called the sped director every day. Unreachable. I felt sure I was being screened. How many other parents of disabled kids were calling him? When I miraculously did reach him, he told me that keeping Jesse home made him a truant and us negligent parents.

I called Mary Somoza, my mentor, who had also dealt with

abusive aides and intractable school administrators. She warned me again to keep every scrap of paper from the school, record every call, and note every development in a diary.

Two weeks later, the team reassembled for the premediation meeting, this time at the special-education offices. In preparation, we had met with an advocate named Jean Vecchiarello from a local agency for the disabled. She made clear to us what we were dealing with. Our school district had no real inclusion. Most kids in wheelchairs were bused out to private, segregated schools or stuck in collaboratives.

I wished I had known of Jean's organization, ARC (Association for Retarded Citizens), before we moved to our town. I had made the grievous assumption that because Massachusetts had a better rate of inclusion than New Jersey, inclusion would not differ from town to town. That was definitely not the case. I now knew, to my sorrow, that sped directors and school administrations could interpret the mandate for a "free and appropriate public education" in the Individuals with Disabilities Education Act with a lot of leeway.

Jean was a veteran of the school wars herself, the mother of a child with Down syndrome, and helped us plan our strategy for the meeting. We would again suggest that Brandy should be Jesse's aide, and we would stress the money-saving features of having an aide whose salary was paid by us. Most schools operated on a tight budget and were looking anywhere to save money; we hoped that under calmer circumstances the sped director and the principal, who had told us he secretly supported us, would agree with the reasoning behind facilitating Jesse's needs and saving cash.

This time the room was less cramped, but the story remained the same. The sped director started by asking if we were prepared to accept the aide. If not, he said, it wouldn't be worth continuing with the rest of the meeting. The meeting ended early.

We had hit a wall. I cursed our luck (and stupidity) at choosing to move to a town a mile away from another town that had full inclusion. I thought about the press. I thought about other parents; we needed to talk to them. The sped director wouldn't tell us who else was in the system: he said he had to respect their privacy. Right.

I called a lawyer. She told me that, legally, Child Protective Services could take Jesse from us if we refused to send him to school.

That night Chris and I sat in a local restaurant we liked because it reminded us of a place frozen in time, Eisenhower's time. Near the bar, a piano tinkled an up-tempo version of "My Favorite Things." Happy Days. Neither of us had any appetite. We picked at our salads, dropping more weight by the minute. We had both lost ten pounds in just three weeks on the Stress Diet. Chris was turning down acting jobs until we resolved the school crisis.

When I told Chris what the lawyer said about Child Protective Services taking Jesse away, he put down his fork and his eyes filled with tears. He made a bridge of his hands to shield his eyes and slowly shook his head. His mute pain and simmering rage made me think about inflicting far worse on the sped director. Who was this person with the power to make our family unhappy every minute of the day? Why couldn't Jesse be safe? Why couldn't our son go to school?

"Chris, take a job. I'll stay here and kill them all," I promised, wildly.

I knew I couldn't do it alone. I had to find the other parents, the ones like us. Was there a tribe of berserker special-needs parents in our school district?

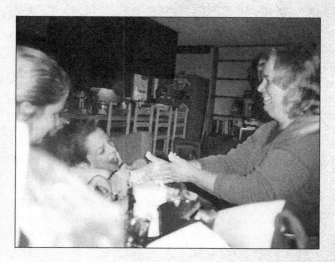

Jess, age seven, building a volcano with Joan Chiampa

I am thankful for my teachers ...
—Jesse's fourth grade journal

CHAPTER TWENTY-TWO

War

April 22, 1996

Dear Parent:

We are parents of a severely handicapped eight-year-old boy who formerly attended [our local] *elementary school. Our attempt at inclusion failed because of the intractability of the school hierarchy, and mostly because of our dealings with* [the sped director]. *We have found him to be arrogant, untruthful and unprofessional.*

We are attempting to form a group of parents to deal with this problem. Are you interested? If so, please call us at [our home number]. *We will arrange a meeting and see what we can do together.*

In unity there is strength!

Sincerely,

Marianne and Chris Cooper

By the time we sent this letter to parents in the district, we had been to mediation. Jesse was still at home, but he had a home tutor for three hours a week. And I had filed a complaint with the Board of Education about the sped director's refusal to remove the abusive aide three weeks after we took Jesse out of school in January, before the mediation. I collected statements in the following weeks from our neighbor Karen; Kelham's mom, Jo; Holly; the director of the eye-gaze computer program at the Boston College Campus School; and Jesse's speech therapist at the learning center.

The sped director replied to the Board of Education about my complaint, saying that the aide had "acted in a professional manner" and that she "was to be commended for her efforts on behalf of Jesse." *Commended.* I pictured Jesse's little fingers bent back as the aide stuffed his arm carelessly into his jacket, Jesse choking and sputtering as the aide crammed a snack into him, Jesse yelling with outrage as the aide discussed his blighted future in front of the class. Last, I pictured doing worse violence to the sped director, my recurring fantasy. The Board of Education responded to my complaint: the aide had not abrogated Jesse's civil rights; at worst she had behaved "unprofessionally" and anyway, they could do nothing while we were in mediation.

I needed to find the other members of the tribe of outraged parents.

Surely Jesse was not the only severely disabled kid in a huge regional school system comprising three towns. Even if there were no severely disabled kids in the local schools, there were kids placed in other systems, like Mass Hospital School or collaboratives. Had they wanted their children included? Had they tried inclusion? I was anxious to meet and talk with these parents.

Jean Vecchiarello gave me an opening when I asked for the names of every parent in our district who had requested an advocate in a dispute with the school from the advocacy center. I had a list of about thirty names. I sent our letter to all of them, and I followed up with phone calls.

Fifteen parents showed up in a room I reserved at our local library. We traded sped director stories, and the heat in the room began to rise. Parents told of their deaf child's hearing aids being taken away as "discipline" at a collaborative, with no action taken by the sped director after their complaints. The mother of a child with rheumatoid arthritis who asked for the services of an occupational therapist was told by the sped director to "wait until she's in a chair" for services. The parents of a high school girl with cerebral palsy told of the sped director saying, "Why should we waste money on these kids? They don't give anything back to society."

That last remark never fails to produce a gasp when repeated, even fourteen years later. The cold, clinical horror of such inhumanity—and this apparently from the sped director, a man who held the futures of disabled children in his hands, a man who was also the deacon at the local Catholic church. I didn't apply a lie detector to these parents that night, but the sheer weight and number of their accusations formed the mortar that held our tribe together.

At that first meeting, a small, balding man with a youthful face joined us. He was Tom O'Brien, our local state representative, and he had set up a table in the adjoining room to meet his constituents and actually do his job—represent the people of his district—*mirabile dictu.* Tom, a former Eagle Scout, took his job seriously and sat behind his little table in the library every month waiting for average citizens to come to him with their concerns. Now he had stumbled into a room full of people who needed his help, and his Scout training kicked in. He became a trusted ally and unwavering friend in the months to come, showing up and speaking at school board meetings in support of our cause.

The tribe decided three things that night: we would organize a parent network in opposition to the sped director; we would attend school board meetings in a group and make the board aware of our dissatisfaction; and we would use the local press to let the public know how their tax dollars were being wasted—far too many special-needs students were being bused out of district to private segregated schools, at great and unnecessary expense.

One parent emerged from this initial meeting who would take the lead in all our future goals and endeavors. That person was Janice Bosecker. She was physically imposing—six feet tall—and carried an intimidating girth that I envied when I pictured her towering over the puny-statured sped director. But she also had a dark and needle-sharp wit; we laughed together on countless late-night phone calls that blew off a little of the pressure pent up from unanswered phone calls and children who were waiting for the basic right to attend school.

Jan's daughter had learning issues and ADD. The district refused to implement Orton-Gillingham and other teaching methods that were employed elsewhere with great success for children with learning disabilities. Orton-Gillingham is a multi-sensory approach that uses phonemics and three basic learning pathways: visual, auditory, and kinesthetic. The method was a proven tool to reduce failure in reading programs for kids with learning disabilities. Most of those kids, including Jan's, had to be bused out of district to private schools that provided this method, at great cost and long travel times for the kids—more than an hour each way for most of them. Other public school districts provided the method with success, but not ours. In fact, one parent claimed that the superintendent had declared that it would be taught "over his dead body" (a fantasy cherished by many of us). There was no rhyme or reason for his stance on Orton-Gillingham. It was incomprehensible, a cruel dictate from a pasha-superintendent who had made our district notorious for its lack of inclusion. The sped director supported his boss on this issue, of course.

Janice ran for regional school board and won that first year. By the end of the year parents of special needs kids had direct input on policies that affected them. It was a regional district, so Janice won in her town, and then another special-needs parent from our group won in our town. Slowly, we began to be heard.

There were articles, letters, and op-eds in the local paper that served our town, then in bigger ones that served the region as the year went on. Six families filed for hearings that year, one of them ours. The "unity is strength" theme was taking hold, and parents who had hesitated to take on the school before were now doing so with determination.

Our negotiations so far had been futile, so Chris and I hired Connie Hilton in April. She was a quiet, determined woman with an encyclopedic knowledge of special-education law and a calm manner in meetings where the tension crackled like an out-of-control California wildfire. She always made sure her seat was next to mine so she could give my ankle a gentle tap whenever my voice rose an octave or two. Connie loved that we called our little nemesis Maria von Trapp and told us, "Thanks. Now I can forever picture him yodeling on an alpine hillside in a dirndl whenever I sit across from him at a mediation."

We loved her dry humor and the compassion that powered her pro bono work for low-income families who were also fighting for inclusion. She had the strawberry blond coloring of a Vermeer subject and projected an unruffled competence in her work. Her own son, also named Jesse, had learning disabilities, and she had done battle with the Cambridge schools to get him the services he needed.

Once Connie came on board, our lives became a flurry of faxes and daily letters. The school district brought on their own lawyer, the formidable Barbara (not her name), who feinted and parried Connie's demands with postponements and "offers" that were merely a series of ever-changing ways to deny Jesse his civil rights. And our connection to Hollywood made us the object of Barbara's sneering remarks.

"Well, they're from *Hollywood*. They should know how to read a *contract*."

The school district's version of *contracts* was varying offers to "include" Jesse by dumping him again. When we requested a special-ed teacher to assist the classroom teacher, the district said that meant Jesse should be in a segregated classroom. But the law stated that he should be educated in the "least restrictive" environment. The school district claimed the right of its own interpretation of "least restrictive environment," and that it was a segregated classroom. But thanks to our mediation, at least Jesse now had the services of a home tutor.

The tutor was Joan Chiampa, who came into our lives that February. I always picture Joan flying through the front door of our raised ranch carrying a sparkle-ended wand, like the slightly ditzy fairy godmother in the Disney movie *Cinderella*. She had the same china blue eyes and a face luminous with innocence. She transferred knowledge to Jesse by sharing her own curiosity and sense of awe at the workings of the world. And she didn't judge. She simply expected Jesse to rise to his own level of awareness, guided by her enthusiasm and delight. And he did.

The benefits that came with mediation were accompanied by stalling tactics in our proceedings against the school district. One afternoon, while I was hammering out a treatment for a screenplay, I took a call from Connie Hilton. She told me about another obstacle the sped director and the administration had lobbed at us, a postponement for no apparent reason except that they were in the position to do it.

My Pavlovian response to the district and their daily chain-yanking was to indulge in my Chub fantasy. Chub was a wise-guy friend of the family who had a soft spot for Jesse. Our son received presents on his birthday every year and an accompanying card signed "Chub and the Boys from the Lake."

Chub was physically, of course, just the opposite—a sinewy

little bantam rooster, a cock of the walk, our local Robin Hood when I was growing up. The *Boston Globe* once did an article on Chub and his good works in the Lake, conveniently leaving out some of his . . . other works. He was old school, the guy who took up the collection for the recent widow, who got the playground equipped, who threw the Christmas party for the neighborhood kids, and the guy who made sure the window of your store was broken if you didn't contribute to the Christmas party. The title of the *Globe* article was a quote from Chub: "Don't Make a Hero Outta Me—It Stinks."

He was my hero, though, because he was a community organizer. And when dealings with Sped Director von Trapp made the vein in my forehead start to throb, I could turn to my Chub fantasy to tamp down the rage.

In the short version of the fantasy, the door to the sped director's office bursts open and Chub plants himself in front of his desk as if he were a towering colossus instead of barely five feet tall. He is accompanied, perhaps, by Starchy and Cuppy, who are much, much bigger. The sped director sputters, half rises, is pushed back into his seat by Chub, who gets in his face.

"The kid, Jesse Cooper, goes to school. Or Starchy and Cuppy here can show you what it's like to be in a wheelchair."

Starchy and Cuppy move in. The sped director screams like a little girl. Close on a pool of urine at his feet. Fade to black over thumping and high-pitched shrieks.

Back in reality, Jesse is stuck at home. But the gloom lifts when I go upstairs. Jesse and Joan are making a volcano for a science project. Brandy is close by, supplying the ingredients. They are covered with flour and baking soda and Jesse is hooting with joy because he is actively involved in making the volcano. Joan and Brandy are laughing helplessly. Joan tells Jesse, "Maybe someday you'll see a real volcano," and I yell, *"Napoli!"* and put on an Italian CD at top volume. Jesse and I dance an improvised tarantella in his chair. If only school could be like this. I am determined to make it so.

That fall, Connie got Jesse back into school part-time in a regular classroom, with Joan acting as his aide. Joan still tutored him at home for ten hours a week. We still didn't have a signed Individualized Education Plan, so Jesse was there on sufferance and could be pulled at any time, at the sped director's whim. Joan was forced to fill out endless paperwork and was harassed by the new principal and vice-principal. The old principal, the one who secretly agreed with us, had left the previous spring. I wondered why, if he knew he was leaving, he didn't follow through with the courage of his secret convictions. Instead, the sped director had begun to insist that Jesse belonged in residential "care," i.e., an institution. And the new principal, an Ichabod Crane look-alike, was the sped director's lackey.

In the middle of the endless negotiations to have Jesse included with a signed and sealed Individualized Education Plan, the school insisted that Jesse be tested by their neuropsychologist, Dr. E. The three-hour test was to be administered at a learning center in the next town. After weeks of delays, a December date was settled upon. Joan accompanied Jesse during the test. Brandy and I waited anxiously outside. Joan finally wheeled Jesse out. She was pale; Jesse was smirky, unaware of the importance of the test.

"Give me a cigarette," she said.

"Joan! You don't smoke!"

At home, over a restorative coffee, Joan told us about the test. Jesse and Brandy were outside building a snowman, Jesse blissfully unaware that he had failed the test.

"He gave him a standard Stanford-Binet IQ test *with no adaptations for his disability!*"

This was roughly equivalent to one of us being asked to read *War and Peace* in ancient Aramaic. Joan described another excruciating part of the test where Dr. E. held up logic-sequence pictures asking Jesse to point to the right answer.

"And whenever Jesse would be just about to point, he would flip over the page!"

Joan was near tears. Had Dr. E. ever actually tested a quadriplegic nonverbal child whose only voluntary movement was a raking grasp and the wavering ability to point? The third part of the test consisted of absurd questions.

"Jesse. Do you *dust* a *dresser?*"

Dust? Mummy didn't dust. Mummy decluttered, Daddy dusted—that was the division of labor in our house. And we called "dressers" bureaus. Or was the doctor asking if Jesse dusted? He didn't. Weirdly, it wasn't a chore I had thought to assign my quadriplegic child. He didn't do windows, either. I asked Joan what Jesse's response had been. She told me he giggled. I'm sure Dr. E.'s "do you dust a dresser" had the same effect on him as *"Twas brillig, and the slithy toves did gyre and gimble in the wabe."* Chris and I, however, were not amused. Jesse had spent three hours in his wheelchair without a break being asked impossible-to-answer questions, which were to be used against him in future negotiations.

I complained to the school board about wasted tax dollars on ridiculous tests. I was sure the sped director was happy because the test gave him the ammunition he needed: he interpreted it to mean that Jesse wasn't up to the challenges of inclusion.

Dr. E., to his credit, hadn't come to any conclusions and had admitted that the test didn't work. Of course, even if Jesse was mentally challenged, and he wasn't, he would still have a right to a "free and appropriate public education," as the Individuals with Disabilities Education Act clearly stated. But our argument with the school still centered on the aide. Connie informed us that we would have a hearing at the Department of Education. We planned carefully for a date when Chris would be in town.

Meanwhile, the parent group was attending every school board meeting and speaking to the press. Janice and I spoke at our local radio station, but I generally tried to avoid speaking to reporters. After the school's lawyer had made gratuitous snippy comments about our Hollywood status, I was nervous about accusations that we were throwing our weight around because of Chris's growing celebrity. The sped director and Barbara, the lawyer, often acted as though I was sweeping into meetings rattling my pearls, with Chris demanding designer water. In reality, they were the ones who grilled Chris about his acting roles instead of talking about Jesse's needs during mediation. Barbara, a tall, angry-looking woman, was a formidable adversary who had faced Connie in many hearings and won some, lost others.

Our little local paper continued to be inundated with angry letters and op-eds from special-needs parents. One of the local reporters, Andrea Doty, wrote a piece about our sped director being "under fire." She wrote that he was on the "hot seat . . . when several parents went public with accusations of poor management of special education services in the district. Several families have hired lawyers to battle the administration on behalf of their children, to get them the services to which the law says they are entitled. One couple has even filed a human rights violation suit against the district." (Guess who.)

The hearings, all six of them, were lined up throughout the school year at the Department of Education. If we won, the school would pay our lawyer's fees, along with their own. So far, it was looking like an expensive year for our district, especially if all six hearings were decided for the parents. And as part of our case, Connie stated that she would file a civil suit for significant money damages for the denial of Jesse's rights to attend school. Our hearing date finally came up on February 12, after months of delay.

We waited outside the hearing room in Malden as the major players in this drama assembled. Connie and Barbara went off to a prehearing conference in another room. Even though the law was with us, we did not feel confident; the hearing officer who was the final decider of our case was a person appointed by the Department of Education, not an independent arbiter. We didn't allow ourselves to think of what would happen if we lost. Where would Jesse go to school? Would we have to move? Where?

Connie joined us, looking upset. We were alarmed. Connie never looked upset. Even when the sped director and Barbara's obfuscation and condescension at meetings gave me the mask of red rage, her serene countenance remained the same.

"What?"

"She was crying," she whispered.

"Barbara?"

Impossible. Impossible to picture this tall, sneering woman of stone in tears.

"She said she had never seen such devoted parents."

"Oh my God! She's possessed!"

Before we had time to posit other theories ("She's been taken over by aliens!"), we were called to take our seats at the conference table in the hearing room.

Before the hearing officer could call the meeting to order officially, the sped director motioned that he wished to speak.

He made a series of proposals in our favor that caused our jaws to drop. They had folded. Completely. Before the hearing even began.

Jesse could return to school for second grade with Joan as his aide in the morning. In the afternoon, she would remain as his tutor at home. This was the compromise we had been hoping for: Jesse would go to school part-time and be tutored at home part-time, and we would have input as to who was his aide, should Joan take another job. At home Jesse could stretch out if his limbs ached from sitting in a chair, and he would benefit academically from the one-on-one tutoring. But he would also experience school with kids his own age and be able to participate in class.

In addition, the school district offered us the services of a speech pathologist who specialized in working with nonverbal quadriplegic children. Lisa Erwin-Miller was a nationally known expert in assistive technology who happened to live locally on the south shore. She would implement a program on Jesse's computer that would allow him to take tests at school, answer questions, and be a part of school presentations. Lisa's program would eventually be the portal that allowed Jesse to access the outside world through his computer.

Why did they capitulate? And why the last-minute drama?

I wish I could say it was because they wanted to do the right thing, that they finally realized that Jesse wasn't getting a "free and appropriate public education" as mandated by law and they wanted to make the system work for him. But I don't think that's why they offered us this bounty on the cusp of the hearing.

I think they must have known they would lose. They surely were feeling the weight of the other five upcoming hearings. They knew that if Connie brought forth the civil suit, we would probably win. And it would cost them money. It would cost them *money.* No matter that Jesse wasn't going to school, that we waited *two years* for justice. It would cost them, so they caved. We never did figure out why Barbara had her tender, teary moment with Connie. Maybe she *was* possessed.

The sped director extended his hand to Chris, who reluctantly shook it. I was not offered his hand, but I doubt I would have taken it had it been offered. A handshake would not erase the sleepless nights, the threatening letters, the loss of half a school year, Jesse's tears, the denial of his basic rights. The paperwork would be up to the lawyers.

The matter was resolved to our satisfaction. That is all our agreement allows us to say.

The following June, a year after the agreement with the

school, at the end of a successful year in second grade, Jesse and Chris were called up to the stage of our local high school. They presented the first annual Jesse Cooper Give Back to Society Scholarship to the teenage girl with cerebral palsy whose parents remember being told by the sped director, "Why should we spend money on these kids—they don't give anything back to society." The sped director sat in the audience watching, because his children were in the school system. But he no longer held the position of special education director. His contract had not been renewed, after a series of contentious meetings with the school board. It felt like sweet justice to see Jesse and Chris up there awarding a scholarship to a disabled student only months after Jesse had been barred from learning among his peers. Now the door was wide open for kids in wheelchairs to come to school. Jesse's ear-to-ear smile lit up the stage.

Jesse would return to that stage in the years to come, to receive his own awards.

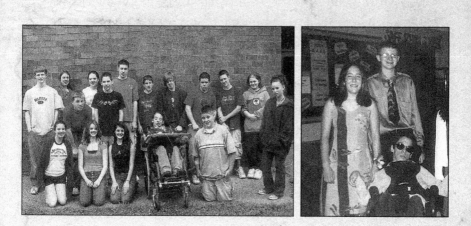

Jess, twelve, with sixth-grade classmates
Jesse, Kyle, and Jamie at their eighth-grade prom

I am always, I am sometimes tough
I am sometimes heroic
I am sometimes tough
I am always, I am always brave
I am always tough
I am sometimes invisible
I am always brave, heroic
I am always, I am sometimes brave
I am sometimes, I am always tough
—*Jesse Cooper*

CHAPTER TWENTY-THREE

Tribute

Jesse was always a warrior boy. He fought for survival in the NICU, pulling out his respirator tube after two weeks, as if to say, "I can breathe on my own now, dammit!" He returned to school while we were still fighting for a valid Individual Education Plan; he knew he was going back to a place where he had been ignored and abused. He had no fear whatsoever.

No hesitancy, no crying, no "behavior." He was helpless, but he wasn't afraid like Chris and I were. Jesse just wanted to be included with his peers. And when he was, when Joan adapted the curriculum so that he did what the other kids did, just differently—he mastered the work and soared like a hawk.

He still had bad days. He still had seizures. He still had bouts of horrifying dystonia, plus the usual coughs, colds, and stomachaches. But in school, he had Joan. And at home, he had Joan as tutor and speech pathologist Lisa Erwin-Miller.

Lisa was a fine-boned, pretty, dark-haired woman who spent hours with Jesse in the makeshift schoolroom we set up downstairs, the sound of her ringing laughter and good-natured coaching pushing Jesse to test his limits. Lisa was as comfortable with nonverbal quadriplegics as a late-night TV host with a voluble guest.

Lisa held the National Conference Program Chair of the U.S. Society for Augmentative and Alternative Communication, and made it possible for all of us to attend their conference on assistive technology in Florida when Jesse was nine. Jesse got so excited when Brandy wheeled him into the exhibit hall he yelled, "Oh shit!" to Brandy. I was thrilled that he said "shit" so distinctly—clearly, he had absorbed the ambience of the Cooper-Leone household. Later that day, Jesse talked computer-to-computer with a nonverbal quadriplegic man who had a master's degree and worked for a software company. Chris and I watched Jesse write sentences to this man and for the first time pictured Jesse in college and beyond, with an actual career.

Lisa taught him the computer tools that truly gave him a voice. She set up a number of boards to help him choose the vocabulary that would ultimately demonstrate how he saw the world. A "feelings" board, for example, would begin with descriptive opposites like: happy/sad, excited/bored. The challenge always was to program the words that would be most interesting for him and give him the widest range of expression, from the mundane request for a drink to the eloquence of a poem. Her interpretation of his word choices began with him pulling the switch. The energy and response time of his "clicking" were additional communication methods he used to indicate whether he liked the word choice or the way a message came out. Lisa told me she could feel his energy when he started communicating through that switch and the computerized speech device. She said that seeing the door of communication open for him was exciting to witness—and something she will never forget.

Jesse could now, for example, learn vocabulary and write reports in English, and even take pop quizzes in school. The teacher would send home the test questions the night before, and Joan or Brandy would put them into the computer. In class, Jesse would take the test along with the rest of the students. There were personal boards, too. Jesse could now tell us if he felt a seizure coming, had a headache, or needed to stretch his limbs. He could converse with new friends, asking them their likes and dislikes.

I could construct "boards" on the computer, but never with the skill of Brandy or Joan. Chris, despite his skills at carpentry and general engineering, was a complete Luddite and technophobe. He acted as if hitting the wrong button would blow up the computer, and he was the butt of family jokes for his terror of the keyboard. He still managed to play computer games with Jesse, coached by the rest of us, but he infinitely preferred swimming, windsurfing, or horseback riding with Jess.

After Jesse was properly tested by Lisa and scored in the ninety-ninth and seventy-fifth percentiles in different parts of the IQ test, there was an expectation of intelligence in school, and that's what changed everything—the perception of Jesse's intelligence. When it was expected of him to do good work, he did, as long as there were supports in the classroom and at home. Every teacher from the second grade on through high school was a willing participant in the inclusion process. His school career after first grade is a long series of triumphs: honor roll every year from middle school on, awards in science, citations for outstanding academic achievement from the President's Education Awards Program. Jesse worked for it. He worked seven days a week, eagerly and joyfully, and he illuminated every classroom he was in. The letter from his sixth-grade teacher, Mrs. Hopkins, is an example of the letters he received at the end of every school year.

Dear Jesse,
I am so fortunate to have you in my class. Your writing
is an inspiration. Your reports are fun and interesting.
Your patience with us is admirable. I love you, Jesse.
Keep growing and loving and learning as you are.
            Your fan,
            Mrs. Hopkins, sixth grade

When Jesse entered seventh grade, Joan Chiampa took a full-time job as a teacher in another school system. His new tutor, Rachel, was a tall, austerely beautiful woman in her twenties, with long dark hair and a New England reserve that Jesse melted in his first session with her.

During that meeting, Brandy and I left Jesse and Rachel alone at the sturdy old dining room table. Rachel was nervous. She read the first question, gave the choices and corresponding letters.

Silence. Jesse listened to the choices and made his decision. The next time through the letters he pulled the switch when it came to his choice. Even though Rachel had been told that Jesse was a good student, she was stunned when Jesse was correct. Jesse continued to be correct more often than not for the next three years Rachel spent as his tutor. He earned honor roll status and Rachel settled in to life in the Cooper house with Jesse.

Rachel learned, too. She learned in many ways that Jesse had something to say. Rachel's serious nature meant that Jesse enjoyed teasing her more than anyone else. One day she was nearly reduced to tears during one of his lessons. I heard Rachel's strained voice asking Jesse to try again, that he just couldn't have gotten every answer wrong. I sat in Rachel's seat, beside Jesse. He looked at me, smirked, and pulled his switch. Every answer was correct. Rachel resumed her seat. Jesse pulled the switch. Every answer was wrong. By then we were all laughing with Jesse, even Rachel.

At the memorial service celebrating Jesse's life, Rachel described Jesse as a voracious learner. Her voice cracking, she said, "When many people first looked at Jesse they saw disabilities and limitations. I grew to see accomplishments and possibilities. Thanks to Jesse, I've learned to always see people first, not bodies."

◼

We got hundreds of letters after Jesse died, some from total strangers, letters so exquisite and moving and painful that their power doesn't diminish when read and reread. For some reason, the letter from his Latin teacher, Mr. Whelton, which consisted of one line characterizing Jesse as "a wonderful boy who had a great talent for Latin," moved me in ways I still don't understand. Perhaps what undid me was this simplicity, the preciseness of his expression, from a man in love with the words of a dead language and the appreciation for a boy who had no way to verbally express language.

Every part of the world Jesse had shared exclusively with others became a little glinting gift to us. The bus driver who simply said that she "remembered him singing on the bus" delivered a clear vision of Jesse singing along with the radio on his way to school, strapped into his chair, happy. It was a way for Chris and me to experience a part of Jesse we never knew when he was alive.

The letters from Jesse's teachers after his death were a validation and a recognition of his daily struggle that strengthened everyone who was a part of it. Death brings hyperbole, flowery and sentimental descriptions of shimmering heavenly vistas when people must write a note of condolence. That goes double for the death of a child. But Jesse's teachers were honest and brave, like he was. They told their real feelings, whether expressed formally or casually. They said he had taught them about love and trust, and to enjoy each day, that he inspired them to live up to the level he set for himself, and that he had given more to them than they could ever give back in return.

Enough. It's starting to feel like I'm channeling some soul-dead movie critic using over-the-top descriptions like "a triumph of the spirit" and "a monumental achievement" and "inspirational" to review my son's life.

When he was in sixth grade, Jesse and I went to Prague to visit Chris filming *The Bourne Identity*. We returned home to Boston via Paris. Jesse kept a journal for the class and reported that Charles de Gaulle Airport was a nightmare of inaccessibility. That was an understatement. After we landed there, the official answer from every airport employee we approached was *"je suis désolé(e)"* when we asked about elevators. Every elevator in the airport was out of commission. Time was growing short for us to make our connection upstairs for the transatlantic flight home; Chris became furious and hefted Jesse's travel chair onto an escalator, muttering his own version of French. But he hadn't counted on the three round concrete barriers at the top of the stairs that prevented us from pushing Jesse's wheelchair through. We fell backward into everyone behind us, like a bad Three Stooges routine. Strangers were screaming, Jesse was laughing, and Chris was horrified.

Jesse's teacher used the escalator incident as a lesson in letter-writing for the class. "They're petitioning to hold the Olympics in France," she told the students. "To whom would you write a letter about what happened to Jesse?"

We have the letters the class wrote. They wrote to the mayor of Boston. They wrote to their senators. They wrote to the Olympics Committee. In the letters, they told about Jesse not being able to get from one place to another easily at Charles de Gaulle Airport. Some letters mentioned elderly people, or parents with babies in strollers. A roomful of eleven-year-olds were now thinking about community, about not just how Jesse gets around, but about old people and young people, and how to make it easier for everyone. Outraged at obstacles like those at de Gaulle happening to someone they knew. Or, as one kid put it:

"Dear Mr. Bush,

Do you know what happened to my friend Jesse?"

Inspirational.

Jesse's scarred brain sent out signals to disrupt his body, his Wicked Witch of the West residing within his skull, hurling lightning bolts at his flailing limbs and sometimes putting a spell on his brain itself, sending it to a frozen, still place at the very moment a poem was trying to be born. But the light that powered the poem, the report, the valentine, the love note on Mother's Day—that light won out over the damaged brain and communicated it to the world around him.

A triumph of the spirit.

The new special ed director who replaced the one that had caused us so much misery wrote to us after Jesse died. "I hope you realize what you and Jesse have done to make our system and our district better. I'd like to think that Jesse's success proves the importance of mainstreaming, working with and listening to families. Even though we certainly still have need for improvement, I hope that the process will continue to improve and be better for other students and that we continue to remind ourselves of Jesse's success when there are challenges."

A monumental achievement.

Jesse, you were always, you were *always* brave.

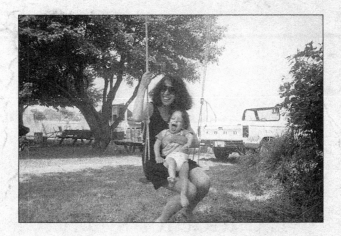

With Jess, age three, on a swing by the bay

My best friend

Out of this world cook!

Takes great care of me

Helps me go places and do things

Exceptional strength

Reads to me

I love you

—Jesse's Mother's Day poem, 1998

CHAPTER TWENTY-FOUR

Ex-Mother's Day

My mother loved oversized, sugary Mother's Day cards with sentimental verses inside, rhyming couplets that induced guilt and at the same time made your teeth ache. Every year I found myself resentfully pawing through pink paper tributes to motherhood at the card store, muttering under my breath.

When I became a candidate for the once-a-year drippy card-and-flowers deal, I let Chris know he was under absolutely no obligation—I wasn't his mother, and Jesse was too young to get the idea behind the day. Maybe when he was four I could deliver a lecture about duped consumer victims to Jesse. And later, I could tell him that Mother's Day had begun with Julia Ward Howe and a plea for peace, so that mothers wouldn't lose their sons in never-ending wars. But Mother's Day got inside

Chris like an alien spore; some combination of surround-sound advertising and free-floating pressure made him go to the store and buy stuff. When Jesse was still an infant I went into his room on Mother's Day and found him in his crib cradling a card in one arm and scented soap in the other. Even though it wasn't from Jesse, I enjoyed the soap. Later, when he was in elementary school, I received teacher-directed cards from Jesse. Nice of them to think of me, but the teachers had written the cards.

But when Jesse mastered the computer, he wrote me quirky poems, which changed everything. My son gave me words, his words, words that were teased out of painstakingly drawn lists, then shaped into thoughts. Words I treasured because they were from Jesse.

Now that I'm no longer a mother, I can ignore Mother's Day, but I'm haunted by words.

So on the day before my second ex–Mother's Day, I got the word *Jesse* tattooed on the inside of my wrist, a semiprivate part of my body that I can look at whenever I want. I'm looking at it now, an indelible filigreed reminder of loss.

Jesse wanted a tattoo. During the summer he was thirteen, we were invited to a backyard barbecue in our neighborhood. We usually saw Forrest, a tattoo artist who hosted the barbecue, or his girlfriend, Rebecca, on our daily walks to the marina. Our dogs played together, Goody dwarfed by their giant Lab. Forrest was goateed and laconic, and Rebecca was a sunny blonde, a Vermont native as robust and healthy as the Vermont Maid picture on maple syrup bottles. At their barbecue, Chris, Jesse, and I were the only unadorned people in a cluster of beautifully embellished skin. Jesse was agog, looking around with a slightly dazed but blissful smile, as if he were spinning on a theme park ride. I asked him if he would like to get a tattoo and he responded with one of his most emphatic clicks. I told him he would have to wait until he was eighteen.

I got the tattoo the year Jesse would have been eighteen.

Chris and I climbed the steep stairs to Cobra Custom Tattoos, incongruously sited among the old-fashioned clapboard-fronted shops on Plymouth's main thoroughfare. Forrest and Rebecca remembered us, though it had been years since they lived in our neighborhood. I told Forrest I wanted a tattoo for Jesse and he showed me a book of memorial tattoos, some of which were huge portraits of the dead meant to span a shoulder or cover a broken heart.

Forrest created a scripted version of Jesse's name with an infinity symbol underneath on a piece of thin, parchment-like paper. It was simple, elegant, and monochromatic black. I approved it—not realizing that the size he showed me was to scale—and he set to work after refusing any form of payment.

The skin is thin on the inside of the wrist, and it was painful getting the tattoo. I welcomed it. Jesse was gone. I wanted to be permanently marked and I wanted it to show. I wanted to flip off other people's happiness with a flick of the wrist, fist raised, a power salute to death.

Chris, silently watching the ritual, had no such impulse. He honored mine, just the same. We're still at the dance together, but he sat this one out. That's okay. He never needed words as much as I did, and I need this word, this symbol of Jesse.

But now, after the rawness of the raised letters has healed, the red defiance has ebbed, and the word on the inside of my wrist is no longer an ashy lament. Today, the tattoo is an exuberant shout, a testimony to Jesse's being in the world, an affirmation of his own wish to proclaim it, and a reminder that I was and will be his mother every day for the rest of my life.

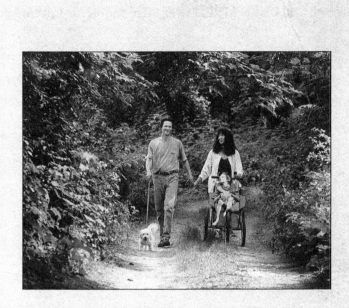

With Jess, Chris, and Goody, 1996

CHAPTER TWENTY-FIVE

Staying Together

I want to be a cowboy's sweetheart
—Patsy Montana

In our earliest days together as a couple, Chris and I slept entwined, inhaling each other like incense. He brought me back to the core of my five-year-old self, the little girl who had lived freely and gloriously in the moment, cocooned in acceptance and love, exploring the world without fear. Chris enabled liberation from the self-doubt and depression of my adolescence and early twenties. He made me laugh like a child rolling down grassy hillsides in summer, giggling an endless spring of bubbling laughter before the source is somehow forgotten in adulthood. I freed something in him, too, a last reserve of shyness, which allowed him to show his full face to the world. I know, too, that I taught him to relinquish the cloistered life of austerity he thought was necessary to pursue acting as a career. Everything about Chris delights me: his essential kindness, his generous soul, his curvy lips, his rare and therefore much-cherished smile, like a seven-year-old's at a birthday party. But this wasn't always so. On our first meeting, he resembled a rabbit sensing a predator, hunched and trembling and poised to dart away.

That night, I consulted my list of hopefuls on the waiting list for acting class, sitting in the risers on our little mini-theater stage in a former carriage house across from Carnegie Hall. I got class free in exchange for managing the list, which was at least six months long. Our teacher, Wynn Handman, was very much in demand, and for good reason: he was the best, a teacher who espoused the clear and direct methods of Sanford Meisner, a founding member of the legendary Group Theatre that included such luminaries of the acting world as Stella Adler and Lee Strasberg. Admission into Wynn's advanced class required an audition, unless a student came in from a midlevel class taught by his affiliates, Bob McAndrew and Fred Kareman.

Now here was Bob, introducing Chris and telling me he would join the class that night, jumping ahead of everyone else on the list. I thought students from the midlevel class went to the bottom of the list. I looked at the supplicant standing there, head down, eyes on the floor. Who was this guy? I bristled, but Bob got his way; Chris joined the class that night. At the next class, he performed a monologue. After class, Wynn commented to me with obvious admiration, "Does that guy know how good he is?"

I was jealous. Most of us in the class were in our twenties, fervently and desperately trying to be good actors. Wynn's approval was the ascension to Mt. Olympus. His criticisms had the opposite effect: I had spent quite a few classes quietly sobbing in the Hadean darkness of our little theater after being told, for instance, "Stop waving your hands around; that's amateur night."

Amateur night. It took all my nascent skills to control my flickering face until I could get to the oblivion of the back row. And Chris was being lavishly praised after his first monologue. I knew he deserved it, but I was still resentful. He didn't even go out for drinks after class with the rest of us! He had none of the easy charm and glib banter that most of the guys in class used to score multiple partners in and out of class. Chris didn't ever make small talk, and he disappeared into the night alone after every class, his trench coat flapping behind him like in the last scene of a film noir.

Then we became acting partners. Partners were randomly assigned according to who was free at the time, having completed either short solo pieces or scenes with others, which spanned several classes. The piece we were given was difficult, a tip of the hat from Wynn, and it would take weeks to finish. It was a scene from Eugene O'Neill's *Mourning Becomes Electra*; Chris and I were to play a nineteenth-century brother and sister, consumed with suppressed incestuous longings. Juicy.

We spent hours together whenever we weren't at our day jobs (carpentry, writing copy for MGM), haunting coffee shops, exchanging life stories—all background for the scene we were working on. I cooked him dinner in my apartment. The bathtub was in the kitchen and my roommate Dale's room opened onto a transom that blasted greasy air from a fast-food restaurant, so it was like sleeping at the bottom of a deep fryer. My room looked onto a vacant lot strewn with litter and discarded furniture. I served spaghetti with clam sauce on a wobbly thrift-shop table and ran out in a frenzy three times for forgotten items (parsley, corkscrew, garlic), while Chris sat bemused and calmly offered to fix the seriously listing table.

I realized why my apartment didn't horrify him when I finally saw his. It was grim, a monk's cell with drab walls and no ornaments, six flights up, in the middle of Hell's Kitchen. He did actually have curtains, but they were sheer and brown, bathing his entire apartment in the color of depression. His scrupulously clean kitchen had only the basics, and his coffee was of the instant variety, off-brand. He had built a loft bed in the tiny bedroom and under that was a desk that looked like he had salvaged it from the street. A knife lay disconcertingly in the middle of the long, dark, creepy hallway into his apartment. I briefly thought that maybe his acting genius was really a cover for homicidal mania, but Chris saw me looking askance at the knife and explained he had been combat-crawling on the floor, acting out his character's Union Army experience. It made sense at the time.

After weeks of rehearsal, improvisation, living and breathing the scene in all our waking and sleeping hours, we finally performed it. Wynn told his afternoon class we "blew the roof off the place." To us, he just smiled and said, "Good work." We were thrilled. But I kept thinking of the moment in rehearsal when Chris gently touched my face, bringing my scattershot focus back to the scene. His never-wavering concentration was a thing to behold. Mine had been shattered when he touched me. A year later, we were finally a couple. It feels now like we moved seamlessly to that place, but I also recall endless middle-schoolish "do you think he likes me" conversations with my best friend, Mary. That's when I wasn't endlessly bugging my roommate about activating his gaydar. No, he assured me, Chris wasn't gay. Then what took him so long? Chris's one-word answer when I posed that question: "Scared." In his Missouri drawl, it came out more like "skeered."

I loved him. I loved that laconic drawl. I loved that he was "skeered"—so was I. He was my archetype. He was the living embodiment of my first crush, the blond cowboy on *Sugarfoot* imprinted on my five-year-old soul, who was always my husband when I played house with my friend Ginny Marzilli. Chris actually knew how to ride horses and had raised cattle on his father's Kansas ranch.

The happy result of Chris's being "skeered" was that when we finally became a couple, we were already friends. And we knew where the drama belonged—onstage, not in what we had together; both of us were veterans of high-drama relationships in the past. All my friends liked him. And Chris passed my movie test: he emerged wet-eyed from Fellini's *Nights of Cabiria,* which I had seen at least sixteen times.

Okay, I loved him. He was The One: my life partner, my soul mate. Now, I thought, *What will drive me insane about him ten years down the road?* What almost indiscernible little foible will be the fingernails-on-chalkboard last-straw moment that sends us both our separate ways? He had a certain unwillingness to engage, a passivity that attracted stalkers. I had seen this for myself: neurotics who had created a fantasy scenario based on Chris's unwavering gentility, mistaking midwestern politeness for encouragement, calling and showing up at his apartment with the persistence of bill collectors. (Even years later, in our little town, we had elderly stalkers drop by the house at all hours after Chris had met and been friendly to them at the local supermarket.) He was so focused on acting, he tended to be absentminded about everything else. And that was the end of my list.

Chris had his own reservations. He was worried that I was too "high-energy" for him. (Polite, as I said.) I would have called it something else. He told me that his career was very important to him. I told him mine was to me, too. We understood each other. He wanted a nonclingy partner. I had never even pictured being married unless I retained my independence. We decided to get married. Very few words were spoken. Very few words were needed.

Chris was the primer, Jesse the tome.

When we decided to have Jesse, we had been married five years. We felt ready. We weren't, of course. No one ever is prepared for the tectonic shift of children changing the heart's terrain. We were both optimistic and scared. I got pregnant immediately and, as an "elderly primagravida," was scheduled for amniocentesis. The genetic counselor explained that we were from such widely differing gene pools, there would be little to worry about.

All you had to do was spend Christmas at my mother's house, and then at Chris's parents', to see just how widely different our gene pools were. Christmas at my house was a huge feast on Christmas Eve, preceded by an afternoon crap game held by the local wise guys at a secret location. Uncle Benny brought Chris that first year. After the feast that night, one of the wise guys' sons, an Elvis impersonator, sat in our kitchen and sang "Blue Christmas," while overexcited kids bounced off the walls and adults sat at the table in the dining room cracking walnuts, eating *torrone,* and arguing loudly. Christmas at Chris's house was midnight service at the Country Club Christian Church and quietly opening presents the next morning with his mother and father, who were both only children. The genetic counselor had an official name for our widely differing gene pools: random mating. "What a great title for a romantic comedy," I told Chris.

Then Jesse was born, ten weeks early.

Once we were aboard the scariest ride in the parenting theme park, we screamed together, tried to balance ourselves around the hairpin turns of Jesse's life-and-death struggle, and giggled in relief when we coasted home. The relief was always temporary before we were once again on the ride. We learned to enjoy the parts where the sun was shining and the wind was in our hair, Jesse tucked between us. We were entwined in a whole new way.

We had a date night at least once a week when Chris was not away on location. Later, when the tender women Bernadette, Suzanne, and Brandy were part of our household, we took the occasional weekend away, usually combining an exotic locale, like Paris or Venice, with Chris's job. I am aware of how privileged we were to be able to do this. We were lucky, but I didn't always feel that way.

"Yeah, well, at least you have fucking room service. I want room service," I yelled at Chris one time after it took me three tries to finally get him on the phone in his L.A. hotel room. My voice had become more strained each time I heard the cheery, forced corporate-speak greeting of the hotel receptionist, probably going on permanent record with her as Chris's harpy wife. I could hear the exhaustion in his faraway voice on the phone; his day had begun sixteen hours earlier. I didn't remember when mine had begun. Jesse had spent the day projectile-vomiting, a violent reaction to the medicine the doctor prescribed for the head lice that came home with him from school. It had taken me three days to figure out he was suffering from fiery, unstoppable itching and that it was why he was so fidgety and irritable. I had screamed at Jesse in frustration and was now exhausted, squirming with guilt and changing bedlinens for the third time that day. I was in the ninth circle of hell, my own head was itching with phantom lice, and Chris was getting room service. And he was getting to be someone else, a character in a film. I wanted to be someone else. Anyone. Someone who didn't want to flay herself alive when she thought of Jesse itching and being unable to scratch and being yelled at for it by his own mother.

There were days like that.

And there were days like this: I finally get Chris on the line and rail about the furnace breaking down, and the kitchen remodel still not finished and the ten inches of snow I had to shovel just to get to the frigging school bus. Chris lets me vent. Then he tells me, "I've been kissing a *guy* for fourteen hours."

Then we both laugh hysterically for the rest of the phone

call. And finally, after we catch our breath, I say, "Come home," and he says, "I'm comin'." But I really mean "I love you," and he means "Yeah, me, too."

Then the little boy that was a part of us was gone forever. In those first surreal days we slept entwined again, but now it was to cling and scrabble and try in vain for comfort. This was the threat that could destroy us—not the challenges we faced in the past, not the fears for Jesse's well-being we had in common or the battles we fought together against the school, not even the flashes of anger over too much time apart or who forgot to get the dog food. The threat to us was of grieving alone, each nursing a private agony, each blaming the other for not feeling exactly what the other was feeling at the same time or in the same way. The threat of bursting apart like seedpods and falling to the ground in separate, dried-out halves, now that Jesse was scattered to the wind and lost to us in this life.

We didn't drown in an eddy of sorrow, but there were days when we just treaded water, waiting for a rescue that never came. There were nights when making love reminded me that I no longer reserve part of myself to be there for Jesse, that I no longer listen for his breathing through the closet that connects our rooms, and in the moment of that recognition, the sharpness of pain blunts the quiver of pleasure. When the tide of sorrow ebbs, we find ourselves again. On those days we cling to each other, but not like desperate survivors. We hold each other like lovers, like partners, like battle-hardened war veterans at a reunion twenty-five years later, in a place where words are no longer needed to evoke the profound memories of the events that shaped us.

Three years later, we've been married for twenty-five years.

Chris carefully hangs a huge picture in our newly renovated bedroom. It's a piece of early-nineteenth-century art that's been crated since his mother sent it to us seven years ago, when she sold the house where Chris had grown up. We had no room in our house to hang it until now, until this new bedroom appeared in place of Jesse's old room. A little girl with long dark hair looks directly at the viewer, unsmiling. She is dressed in black, and holds a jump rope limply in her hand. She looks uncompromising and vulnerable, as if her privileged life holds some secret sorrow. I say, "Hey, Chris, she looks like me."

"Yeah, and I've loved her all my life."

He says it offhand, like someone chewing a blade of grass.

Before I can swoon, he adds, helpfully: "And she has your underbite."

I push him onto the bed and we tumble over and over, laughing like children rolling down a hill in summer.

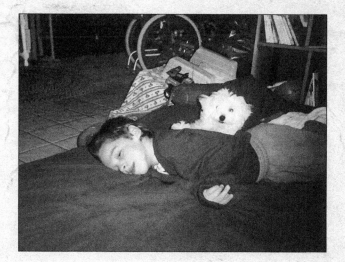

Jess, seven, and Goody

"Goody feels furry, tickly, soft and cottony ..."
—*Jesse Cooper*

CHAPTER TWENTY-SIX

Lucky and Frenchy

Two bedraggled faces peered at me from the adoption Web site Petfinder.com. Lucky Dog, a bichon frise, was three years old, and French Fry, a bichon-poodle mix, was two. They had been captives of puppy mills, nefarious dog prisons that kept dogs under appalling conditions and bred them until they died. Together they called to mind woeful street orphans from a hundred-year-old daguerreotype. Lucky looked like a tough guy and the protector of Frenchy, his pitiful sidekick. They came as a duo—no separate adoptions allowed. I wasn't a prospective adopter; I was just looking. And looking. I kept going back to the site and staring at those two hurt creatures.

Lucky looked just like Goody, but with an attitude. After the surgery to remove the Not-Jesse, I was the semiwalking wounded, recovering on my daybed, watching reality shows to see if they bore any relation to my current reality, which seemed more like a particularly disturbing episode of *The Twilight Zone*, and visiting Petfinder when I could drag myself over to the computer.

Goody was a prince among dogs, raised in the warmth of our family pack. When Jesse blurted out his request for a dog to Santa, time constraints and ignorance made us do a terrible thing: we bought Goody from a pet store. We didn't know then that we were supporting the puppy mills that torture animals like Lucky and Frenchy.

I showed the orphan picture to my husband. Chris was noncommittal, but there was no mistaking the softening around his eyes. We became prospective adopters. Three recommendations, one of them from our veterinarian, and a home visit were required. The day of the home visit, Chris stuck around long enough to meet the woman vetting us, and then disappeared on an "errand." I looked at pictures of her Pomeranians (nine of them), agreed to subscribe to *Bark* magazine, and tried to reassure her that we wanted the dogs. She asked about the portrait of Jesse in our living room, and I told her he was our son, that he had been disabled, and that he died. She began to cry.

"Then you'll know how to nurture these dogs, because you had a special-needs son," she said.

I have a terrible poker face. My acting teacher was always pointing out that on film I would look like a cartoon character if I didn't learn to rein in my overly mobile features. I have no idea what registered on my face to the interview lady, but inside I felt like a multiple personality. One identity, the Marianne who grew up in the Lake, took a drag of her cigarette and said,

"Yeah, right, lady, raising my kid was just like raising a dog." Another character, St. Marianne the Merciful, agreed with the interview lady: "That's what these dogs will need, unconditional love, and that's what we gave Jesse." The third identity, the Pragmatic Marianne, was the one that I hoped was dominating my facial features. That identity wanted to smile politely, get through the interview, and get the dogs.

We passed the interview, somehow.

After signing impressive-looking contracts (how would they enforce them?) and promising never to kennel the ex-prisoners, we drove to Connecticut to rescue the dogs. It was a soft June day, four months after Goody died, four months after the surgery, thirty months since our son had died.

On the first day, I took stock. They weren't housebroken. They didn't know their names. They shrank from us, so no leash was possible. I thought, What if they bolt? and pictured the formidable interview lady checking up on us, only to find we had allowed Lucky and Frenchy to be crushed by a school bus on their first day of freedom. That horror scenario propelled me to full alpha dog mode; I stood tall (as tall as I could), barked out their names in a commanding voice, and they followed me outside, jolted into action by the sound of my voice. They ran, tottering like elderly little men on walkers, their legs stiff from a life encaged.

I blinked back tears and herded them into our enclosed pool area. Their true dog selves emerged; they began cavorting and chasing each other. Lucky, the madder of the two, careened around a corner and fell into the pool. Chris heard me scream and jump in after Lucky, and stood on the deck above the pool, laughing, as he watched me haul myself out of the water, hampered by clothes that now weighed a ton. Lucky pranced off, unperturbed and ungrateful for my lifesaving heroics. Chris brought me a towel, still laughing. In the days to come, we laughed a lot. Our laughter was creaky from disuse, like Lucky's and Frenchy's legs.

It's now a year later. They've commandeered the comfy chair. They're housebroken, they know their names, and they walk on leashes (Lucky bites his). Frenchy nudges my leg, asking for caresses. Lucky still runs away if I even glance at him and sleeps with one wary eye open. He's my favorite because he's both dauntless and terrified, and reminds me of me. In bursts of bravery he'll stretch himself forward, quickly lick my hand, then bolt. I stalk and capture him to put him in my lap and pet him.

"You heal me and I'll heal you," I whisper.

He jumps down, turns around, and dog-smiles. He keeps his wary eye on me.

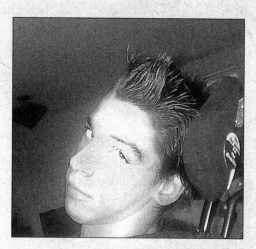

Our last photograph of Jesse, age sixteen

I am a poet
I speak through my poems
And people listen
—*from Jesse's last poem, "I Am"*

CHAPTER TWENTY-SEVEN

Finding Jesse

When I try to find Jesse every day, I am not expecting the gasp-producing, transcendent Madonna-and-Son reunion in the Piazza Garibaldi. Such bliss is meted out only in seconds of unconsciousness when I meet Jesse, hold him, kiss him in dreams that are really visits from him. I look for him in the sky but the hawk isn't there as often as I need to see him.

Jesse told me in a dream visit, "I'm always with you." I take him at his word and talk to him. I ask him to send me songs sometimes when I'm alone in the car, just another of the many shifts in sanity in my life without Jess, like talking to myself and addressing inanimate objects out loud. Anyway, he does send me songs when I turn on the radio: "You're In My Heart." "(Your Love Keeps Lifting Me) Higher and Higher." "You Learn." And I feel a frisson of contact for that moment. But the hunger for touch is abated only temporarily in the seconds of dream-visit bliss. I don't try to find that bliss every day because the touch we shared was only one part of what was Jesse, alive.

It is the giving part I miss, the feeling of giving to Jesse without expectation of anything in return. And now that's how I experience Jesse in the fullest way, in the giving. By giving I don't mean to charities, though I know he would appreciate the foundation in his name that helps other kids with disabilities to go to school. I mean the giving of myself to others in less tangible ways, the sympathetic ear, the small thoughtful remembrance, the acknowledgment of other people's joys and sorrows. That's exactly what I don't want to do. I want to stay inside and be alone. I want to wander the rooms of my house blankly, like a confused spirit trapped between worlds. But I can't find Jesse that way.

I try to use my mother-warrior skills to train future warriors and to slay the bitterness and loss of hope in my own treacherous heart. I talk to mothers who have babies like Jesse. They are afraid, angry, desperate. Like I was. I hold their babies and I tell them they will have joy, that they have a teacher. They don't always believe me. I don't blame them. I am aware that I sound like a refrigerator magnet. They see work, unending work, and years of fighting ahead. And they see my work as over. But it's not. I'm still trying to find my son.

Chris and I take part in a circle dance that brings us somehow winding back to Jess. It starts with us, giving to each other. If I interrupt my own dazed stumbling to touch Chris, if I roll out the aches in his shoulders from a day of burning deadfall, I suddenly find Jesse. I am hurtled back into a moment in time when I am rubbing Jesse's shoulders and I can feel his hon-eyed skin and hear his languid click, his *yessssss,* and I can see his long-lashed lids quivering, fighting sleep. Jesse is present, found, invoked by giving. To be present in the world, the world without Jesse, that's the hardest thing. But it's the only way to find him.

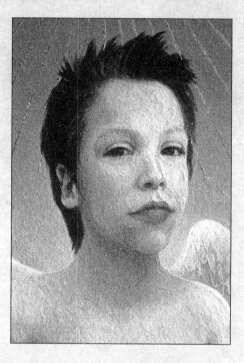

Portrait by Adrienne Crombie,
commissioned when Jesse was four

THANKSGIVING

My family is fancy

I give you joy.

I give you love.

I give you care

Hope

We celebrate.

At Thanksgiving I feel love.

I thank, I give.

—*Jesse Cooper*

Acknowledgments

For years, whenever I attempted to write prose I felt the weight of Colette on one shoulder and James Joyce on the other. Colette always gave me a Gallic shrug of dismissal. Joyce snickered nastily. Jesse changed all that, and telling his story helped me unload those two and sit at my computer, unburdened by impossible comparisons.

Heartfelt thanks to Grub Street, a Boston writers' group that provides workshops for the writer wishing to explore every form of the written word. Alexis Rizzuto's memoir workshop relieved me of my irrational fear of prose after years in the world of screenplay. My gratitude to Alexis for her kind and unending encouragement, and to the members of the two workshops in which I began to write this book. Particular thanks to Robin Grace, Susan Klein, and Carrie Normand, who slogged through every chapter with me until the end, and whose carefully written critiques encouraged me to pay attention to detail and to always go deeper. Thanks also to Karen Dempsey, who offered the same care and attention via e-mail, as well as Mary Granfield.

Love and deep gratitude to the people who knew and saw Jesse in his life and helped me find him again for this book: my sister, Lindy; my brother, Michael; and Jesse's cousins, as well as Brandy Sliney, Holly Dolben, Joan Chiampa, Rachel Bird, Jo Stephenson, Lynne Bailey, Karen Wheble, Connie Hilton, Nancy Savoca, Mary Portser, Janet Tashjian, Maria Manduca, Dale Carman, Ann Brown, Dorothy Aufiero, Patty Ross, Mary Somoza, Dr. Elizabeth Thiele, Dr. Sandy Helmers, Lisa Erwin-Davidson, Kathy Spicer, Maureen Clark, Emmy Clarke, John Sayles, and Maggie Renzi.

I want to also acknowledge readers Dr. David Ryan and his wife, Carol, for their support, as well as Michael Lazo and Maureen Hancock.

Many thanks also to Colleen Mohyde, my agent, who has shown an interest in this book since it evolved from a raw essay published in the *Boston Globe* three months after Jesse died. I am very grateful for her kind encouragement and guidance, not to mention the hours we've spent together giggling over the parochial school atrocities of our similar girlhoods.

My stunned gratitude to Priscilla Painton and David Rosenthal of Simon & Schuster for their fierce championing of Jesse's story. I also thank the extraordinarily gifted Michael Szczerban, who used his bountiful talent to help shape this manuscript into the book it became. There is no one I'd rather parse words with, and I am already missing our time together working on Jesse's story.

Finally, my love and gratitude beyond measure to the unnamed members of the community who embraced Jesse and his story both during and after his life.

The Jesse Cooper Foundation

The Jesse Cooper Foundation supports inclusion in public schools through the Federation for Children with Special Needs, adapted sports for disabled kids through AccesSportAmerica, and the disabled orphans of Romania through Romanian Children's Relief.

For more information, write:

Jesse Cooper Foundation
P.O. Box 390
Kingston, MA 02364

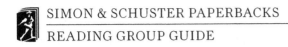

Jesse

Introduction

Jesse Cooper was an honor-roll student who loved to windsurf and write poetry. He also had severe cerebral palsy and was quadriplegic, unable to speak, and wracked by seizures. He died suddenly at age seventeen. In *Jesse: A Mother's Story*, Jesse's mother, Marianne Leone, shows readers that despite challenges along the way—including her struggle to integrate Jesse into the public school system—life with Jesse was more rich and joyful than anyone could have imagined. In his short lifetime, Jesse lived life to the fullest and brought unbelievable happiness to everyone he met. *Jesse* is a heartbreaking, spirited, and poignant memoir, in which Marianne writes passionately about her family's journey—the hope, challenges, grief, and love.

Discussion Questions

1. *Jesse* is filled with humorous scenes, such as when Jesse kicks a monk who is trying to bless him. Discuss the tone of the book and how Marianne was able to infuse her story with moments of levity and hope. Were you surprised by the comical moments in the book?

2. From a struggling actress in Hell's Kitchen to a disability advocate in small-town Massachusetts, Marianne becomes a very different person by the end of the book. How does she change throughout the course of Jesse's life? Can her transformation be solely attributed to Jesse, or are there other factors at work? What did Jesse teach Marianne?

3. How do Jesse's poems provide insight into his thought process and his perspective of the world? How did he perceive himself and the challenges he faced? Which of his poems affected you the most? Which one provided the most insight into who he was as a person?

4. At Jesse's memorial service, Marianne says that "parents of disabled children are 'touched by the Divine.'" (pg. 11) What do you think it means to be "touched by the Divine?" How have you been "touched by the Divine?"

5. Jesse writes, "Courage is like one ant trying to cross a roaring stream. It may seem impossible but you have to try." (pg. 135) How does Jesse demonstrate courage throughout his life? How does Marianne encourage this character trait in her son, and how does she embody this spirit herself?

6. When Jesse is in first grade, Marianne exchanges daily notes and journals with his teacher. Despite her growing frustration, she says, "I continued to write cheerleadery rah-rah responses to Jesse's teacher's misspelled messages." (pg. 177) Why does Marianne initially alter her personality when dealing with Jesse's teachers and aides?

7. Why is Jesse's school so resistant to Marianne's efforts to improve Jesse's experience in the classroom? Were you frustrated by the difficulties Jesse faced in school?

8. Who does Marianne turn to in difficult times? How does she create and maintain her support system? Who are the people in your life that you turn to for support?

9. Marianne is a self-described "rageaholic," and even experiences blackouts at times when she is extremely angry. What incites her rage the most? How does she use her rage to her advantage, and when does it hurt her?

10. Throughout Jesse's life, several female caregivers enter the Cooper household and teach, tutor, and help Jesse. Describe the bonds that form between Jesse and the women

and between Marianne and the women. How do these women affect the family?

11. Despite the difficulty of parenting a child with disabilities and the physical separation that was often required for Chris's acting jobs, Marianne and Chris's marriage remains strong throughout the book. How is their relationship affected by Jesse's disability? How do they handle the stresses that come along with fighting for their son's right to attend school?

12. Marianne says that she "sees" Jesse in the strangest of places, from an old man praying in Naples to a hawk flying in the sky outside the hospital. When and how does Marianne see Jesse? Why does Jesse take the various forms that he does?

13. In Jesse's last poem, he wrote, "The world is my book / I hear all its voices." (pg. 29) What do you think he meant by that? How does Jesse communicate with the world, and how does the world communicate with him?

Enhance Your Book Club

1. Get involved! Host a charity event—bake sale, yard sale, or 5K run—and donate the money to a charity, like, www.cerebralpalsy.org, www.ucp.org, or find the parent-to-parent disability org in your state. You can also donate to the Jesse Cooper Foundation. Visit www.marianneleonecooper.com for details.

2. Spend an afternoon volunteering with children who have disabilities or any other cause about which you feel passionately. Visit to www.volunteermatch.org, www.serve.gov, or www.dosomething.org/volunteer to locate volunteer opportunities in your community.

3. Marianne becomes an advocate for Jesse and his right to attend school like any other child. Discuss a time in your life when you felt so passionately about something or someone that you were willing to do whatever it took to achieve your goal.

4. Although he often struggled to communicate verbally, Jesse's writing is full of life. His poems display a wealth of emotions and keen observations of the world around him. Write a poem about something you have struggled with in your life and share it with your group.

Author Questions

In the acknowledgments section, you talk a little about the writing process for *Jesse*. What made you decide to write the book? Was it difficult to share your story? Did you ever want to quit, and if so, what made you keep going?

I wrote an essay for *The Boston Globe* about three months after Jesse died, and the book grew out of that essay. At the end of the essay I quoted Jesse's first poem, "Inside/Outside" which had the lines "On the inside I speak," and "On the outside I give." In the closing lines of the essay, I wrote, "So I'll walk on the inside and give on the outside. But I can't be mute. I think Jess would understand that I have to give sorrow words."

"The grief that does not speak whispers the o'erfraught heart and bids it break" (Shakespeare). Shakespeare gave voice to the human condition better than anyone. The pain of loss compels the writer to "give sorrow words" to deal with that pain.

The only difficult part of sharing this story was the reliving of the battle to have Jesse included in his local public school. I felt again the despair and rage at the unfair way Jesse was treated, and anger at my own incompetence and slow learning curve in this brave new world of special education.

What made me keep going was the desire to share with others the impact this nonverbal child had on so many people around him. Despite the agony of reliving his struggles, I also experienced the utter joy of Jesse's company in writing this book and that helped me keep going.

Can you describe the responses you have received from the book? Has anything surprised you?

I have received scores of heartfelt letters both via snail mail and as e-mail comments on my blog at www.marianneleonecooper .com. Many have been moved to enclose a donation to the Jesse Cooper Foundation. So many of the readers who wrote me (and they were mostly mothers) talked about snatching precious moments of time while waiting for a nurse to arrive or checking to see if their child was still breathing. They told me how much this book and Jesse's story resonated with them. These letters moved me to tears and brought me instantly back to my own stolen minutes of writing time when I was acting and writing and being Jesse's mom. I got a letter from a thirteen-year-old girl who went to Jesse's school and whose teacher had directed the class to read a book about a person with a disability. She said she wished she could "hand the book to every person in the world so they could know about Jesse." More than one person described the book as a "love letter" to my son, which made me happy. The educators and therapists who wrote gave me hope, especially the ones who said they would never look at a child like Jesse in the same way again. And there were even funny letters, like the one that told me my book should come with a warning label: "Caution! My son's a charmer and you will be in love with him for the rest of your life."

From your upbringing in the Catholic church to your decision to teach Jesse about all the world's religions, can you talk about your faith and the role it played in your life with Jesse?

Jesse was my spiritual teacher. I learned about unconditional love from him. I don't know if you could exactly call that having a faith, unless you think of it as having faith in the power of unconditional love to transform us all into our best selves. I am, in the words of Jackson Browne "a heathen and a pagan on the side of the rebel Jesus."

What is your happiest memory of Jesse?

There is no one happy memory frozen in time. My memories feel more like navigating a river that flows from the sweet trill of Jesse's giggles to the silky feel of his skin to his smile of triumph at doing well on a school test—that's on a good day. On a bad day, the river freezes over and I'm trapped in the memory of finding him dead.

How are you continuing to work with parents of children with disabilities and cerebral palsy? Have you continued to work with the school district in your area? What changes have been made since Jesse?

For the seventeen years I was Jesse's mother advocating for his inclusion, I was also a writer and an actress. I honestly think that in my case it made me a better mother to keep a part of myself that was not only Jesse's mother. I continue to act when I can, and to write. But I am not a full-time advocate. I hope that this book serves as an inspiration to educators. I am motivated by the words of a teacher who wrote, "I will never again look at a child like Jesse in the same way after reading this book." I plan to visit universities and talk to future teachers, therapists, and social workers about inclusion and working fruitfully with parents to achieve their disabled child's goals at school.

What advice would you give to parents of children with disabilities who are feeling discouraged and frustrated with their schools or doctors?

Turn on the radio to your favorite music, blast it, and dance with your child in or out of a wheelchair. When they laugh, use that laughter as fuel to keep going. Remember that you are your child's strongest advocate. Seek out the parent-to-parent organization in your state (every state has one; in Massachusetts it's the Federation for Children with Special Needs) and ask for help from other parents who've been there. Meet with them and take strength from your unity.

Other than your husband, who was the person you leaned upon most while Jesse was growing up? How did you maintain such a strong network of support around you at all times?

Both my and Chris's family, though geographically distant, were always there for us. Also our friends, who were mostly single and childless with the exception of one couple, but all of them were willing to babysit Jesse so we could have a night out. We made sure to have a date night every week, even if it was just a quick dinner in a local diner. When Bernadette, Jesse's first wonderful nanny, came on board, we were able to travel more easily and even had our first weekend away alone together. Suzanne was with us only a year, but her warmth and kindness helped our transition to a small New England town. Then Brandy was with us for ten years, until Jesse died. She was like a big sister to Jess and a daughter to us. We are still in close contact with the circle of caregivers and therapists who were part of our family. I don't know how to explain this except to say that Jesse's light drew us in and the memory of that light keeps us together.

Can you share more about the Jesse Cooper Foundation and the work that you are doing now?
The Foundation is really very small, and so far only in Massachusetts (and Romania!). We receive small contributions from people who've read about us, and Chris and I are the biggest contributors. I am tithing myself ten percent of the proceeds from this book for the Foundation. It would be bigger if it were my full-time pursuit, but both Chris and I are mainly actors and writers.

The Jesse Advocacy Fund administered through the Massachusetts Federation for Children with Special Needs helped twenty-one low-income, non–English speaking families include their disabled children last year by providing advocates to assist the parents. The Jesse Cooper Foundation helps the Romanian Children's Relief Foundation, specifically the program which supports the disabled children and teenagers' health conditions and the facilitation of these children away from institutions and into foster and group homes. The Romanian Childrens' Relief Foundation also provides therapy, educational, social, and recreational activities, and works to enhance the awareness and acceptance of disabled children in the community. AccesSportAmerica specializes in windsurfing, kayaking, rowing/sculling, outrigger canoeing, surfing, water-skiing, and kite sailing, as well as rock/wall climbing, tennis, cycling, and soccer. Programs are designed to promote each person's highest physical and athletic potential while cultivating social and emotional well-being. The exhilaration inherent to each sport is just a part of the experience which fosters positive change in function and fitness as well as attitude and expectation for a life lived with a disability. Athletes, through individually developed programs, experience a series of unparalleled accomplishments through mastery of balance, coordination, and fear. Over 1,500 athletes participate annually year round in Massachusetts.

What is the most important thing that Jesse taught you?
Patience, and the ability to look beyond the superficial. Jesse taught me to go deeper, face fear and develop the focus of a warrior. I will be grateful for those gifts for the rest of my life.

What is the one thing you would like readers to remember about Jesse?
I think Jesse's poems showed how he wanted to present himself to the world. "On the inside, I speak." "I am a poet. I speak through my poems / And people listen." And in his sixth grade autobiography he wrote, "The most important lesson I can teach is to see people for what they can do and not for what they cannot do." I think he would be most pleased by the number of readers who saw him as a typical, mischievous teenage boy.